四季健康法 Staying
Healthy
With the
Seasons

Examples of imbal in emot → physical manif
+ grief   chr. lung prob

四季健康法

Staying Healthy With the Seasons

Elson M. Haas M.D.

CELESTIAL ARTS
BERKELEY, CALIFORNIA

Cover painting by Marshall Peck, III
Art Direction by Neil Murray and Abigail Johnston
Illustrations by Richard Moffett and Pam Twachtmann
Calligraphy by Primrose
Composition by HMS Typography

The illustrations on pages 15, 28, 29, 37, 48, and 168 are available printed on T-shirts for adults and children, and the illustrations on page 48 are printed on sox. These items are available from

Harvest Health Unlimited
P.O. Box 427
Fairfax, CA 94930

The author would like to thank Health Harvest, Leslie Arwin and The Medical T-Shirt Company for the use of this artwork.

Celestial Arts
P.O. Box 7327
Berkeley, California 94707

First Printing, April 1981

Manufactured in the United States of America

Library of Congress Cataloging in Publication Data

Haas, Elson, M. 1947–
Staying healthy with the seasons.
1. Climatology, Medical.   2. Health.   I. Title.
RA793.H3   613'.13   80-69469
ISBN 0-89087-306-2 (pbk.)

11   12 — 90

To my dear friend, Bethany S. ArgIsle,
for your inspiration, vision, and perseverance
which have given form to this book.

To Hal Kramer and Barry,
for your support and faith.

And to the many other people and spirits
who helped along the way—

Thank you.

Contents

四季健康法 Staying
Healthy
With the
Seasons

Whoever wishes to investigate medicine
should proceed thus:
In the first place, consider
the seasons of the year
and
what effect each of them
produces

HIPPOCRATES

Introduction

DURING the latter stages of internship and afterwards while working in several general medical, pediatric, and drop-in clinics, I grew more and more aware that I did not have answers or helpful treatment for many people. In fact, I had to search my repertoire to find some acceptable thing to do for my patients, who were expectantly waiting for the doctor's action.

Many vague complaints, lingering aches, or acute "viral syndromes" seemed to fill the clinics; a complete history and physical exam, x-ray and laboratory tests revealed only findings "within normal limits." I often had to leave the patient with, "Well, everything seems to be fine." Prescribing rest and giving reassurance seemed to be my main treatment. The normal testing and reassurance seemed to allay the fears which many people had that some external disease might attack and kill them, or even worse, mutilate and leave them functionless. The patient often seemed to be seeking an outside God-like power to tell her or him that all was okay; the doctor had to fill that role for the moment.

Much health difficulty seemed intertwined with life's daily stresses, tension in family relationships, and worries about jobs or money. All those fancy diseases I had heard about in medical school were few and far between, and I had little chance to use the medications with which I had been taught to treat. In fact, I saw many medication-caused problems. Some-

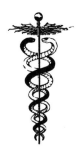

thing just wasn't right. I was reminded of the Hippocratic Oath I took at medical school graduation, "I will use treatment to help the sick according to my ability and judgment, but I will never use it to injure or wrong them. I will not give poison to anyone though asked to do so. . ."

My own judgment was telling me that there were answers and understanding beyond these accepted interpretations of disease and treatment. Thus in late 1973, I went to work in a setting where I could seek a deeper and more helpful understanding of illness and health. I began working with two other doctors at a clinic in Northern California which was exploring the benefits of various body therapies, herbal medicine, and biofeedback, when combined with traditional Western medicine.

At the time I arrived, my two new colleagues were in the middle of a research study on the use of high-frequency sound in acupuncture treatment, along with relaxation techniques and the use of mental imagery, that is, the patient's visualization of the body healing its own problems. It was not only very interesting, but the results I began seeing were quite impressive, even mind-boggling. They just didn't fit into my Western framework. But according to scientific method, if the results are not as predicted, one should reevaluate his hypothesis. So I began reevaluating things.

My move to live in a country setting brought even more alive my interest in disease prevention, health enhancement, and the root causes of illness. All these were important in my choice to use and observe the effects of nature's non-invasive remedies on our well-being.

My outlook moved from, "Oh, that flu is going around," "It's a virus," or "It was an accident," to a sense that *we* may actually create or draw to us every experience or illness manifested so that we may learn and grow from it. Illness represents an invitation to change. I see this deeper understanding as very important. Of course, this does not deny the existence of microorganisms or accidents, but it gives us a different focus. Creating a healthy body and being in harmony with nature and with one's own inner guidance will help prevent infections and other mishaps.

In this book, I explain many approaches and specific advice to clear the body of its problems, and ways to open up to and pursue *health*. These are not proposed as treatment plans for any ailment, though there is much helpful information herein.

Much of this information is best classified along the lines of belief systems, which I call the "intuitive sciences." They seem as appropriate now as they have for thousands of years. Much of this information is not, however, proven under the scientific method, such as the use of specific studies with control groups.

If you or your friends need treatment for a specific illness, you would do best to seek treatment from your doctor/helper, as the *interpersonal exchange* is vitally important to the healing process. My suggestions are from firsthand experience of both new and ancient healing methods that work. The key lies in your getting in touch with your own self, and in seeing both the process of disease and the process of healing as a useful means of learning about yourself.

In my practice, I combine diagnosis, treatment, and education, or really "re-education." I do a complete medical evaluation at all levels—physical, emotional, mental, and spiritual —then create *with people* a specific program which will help rid them of their illness, improve their general health, and prevent the return of any difficulties. (Very optimistic? Of course!)

I call this a "creative health program." The overall objective is to find out where you are and where you wish to go, and then work on how to get from here to there. It involves an initial extensive history and complete physical exam, and any necessary x-ray or laboratory tests. In a second deeper session the body systems are tested for stress, weakness, and congestion. I use my Western training as well as my background in Chinese medicine to help me understand the body state. Each therapeutic program is individual and usually contains some lifestyle changes in giving up certain habits, finding a more suitable diet, even prescribing certain foods or herbs which may help cleanse, build, and/or balance body systems. Often we may have therapeutic sessions for physical and mental relaxation and emotional balance, to help achieve greater daily health. I also employ a specific therapy which I helped develop, called *sonopuncture,* the use of sound vibrations via ultrasound or medical tuning forks in acupuncture treatment. This has a very relaxing and balancing effect. Ultrasound is transmitted by a small machine which emits, via a low electrical current, one megacycle of sound vibrations into the body through a quartz crystal contained in a portable applicator head. Tuning forks have specific frequencies of vibration more attuned to the audible and physical range of the human species, and each fork's frequency creates a specific note which is also associated with a certain color.

Obviously, there are a variety of therapeutic modes discussed here. This may be confusing at first, but like most things, the more you work with it, the simpler and clearer it becomes. It's all connected!

It is important to incorporate all things into our medicine which can aid in understanding illness and deciding treatment, focusing more on education and prevention. But this process must begin with yourself. Much health improvement takes real work on your part, and daily care. Healing is a process, not a destination. Illness is usually not imposed on or separate from us. It is more our own lack of self-control, moderation, and direction which endangers our health, though environmental and economic factors are certainly concerns.

When we are in transition, or it appears that our world is dissolving, let us pay attention to what we feel within ourselves. This awareness is vital to health. The understanding of who we are, and what we are feeling and doing in our lives, and then living and acting with this clarity of awareness, will keep us well.

You each have an inherent life program, an individual purpose as part of the greater purpose; and your individual needs often reflect this. Disease comes from being out of touch with your program, but the harmony between your inner direction and outward action will bring you happiness. Let your needs surface, and you will become aware of your real goals, immediate and long-range. You will then be able to create new plans for your health and life and give birth to your new self.

Staying Healthy with the Seasons really began in 1975 when I started a seasonal newsletter for the local people of the town in which I practiced. The response and encouragement which followed those early writings stimulated me to expand the concepts and information into what you find here.

My basic premise is that there is a two-way communication between man and nature, and that this affects both your inner harmony and growth and your physical well-being. Closely following the Chinese philosophy of health and illness, *Staying Healthy with the Seasons* explains the Chinese Law of the Five Elements—Fire, Earth, Metal (or Air), Water, and Wood—and how this system relates to specific seasons of the

"Know matter what. . .
We grow.
Know matter what. . .
We think we know
We grow!"

B.S. ArgIsle

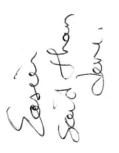

year, organs in the body, and experiences of activity, emotion, color, and flavor.

The concrete applications of the Chinese system of medicine and its use in our everyday health in the light of Western medical knowledge are of particular concern. For example, times of seasonal change are important as reorganizational periods, and are times for increasing self-awareness and looking at life priorities, but are also times of greater stress, and thus of potential illness or physical difficulty. Your adaptation to these changing seasons is vitally important to your continuing good health. For example, just as in spring, you may find yourself engaged in new projects, new friendships, and more activity during the growing sunlit days, your life during the autumn may be evolving in the opposite direction, reflecting decreasing sunlight and longer night hours. At this time, you may be back at work or school after a summer vacation, and feeling more disciplined and focused on yourself; you may work at completing plans and projects that you began in the spring and summer.

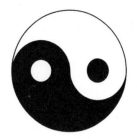

Staying Healthy with the Seasons also incorporates the use of diet and exercise and how these could change through the year for best results. Food both creates your body and serves as your fuel. Depending on your climate and activity, your optimum foods will vary in content and quantity. Good dietary suggestions and eating habits for a long, healthy life are emphasized. Exercise and activity levels also change with the season and weather. Daily movement is important to loosen muscles and joints, as is regular aerobic exercise to stimulate deep breathing, circulation, and sweating. There are many suggestions for ways to relax and alleviate stress.

Other aspects of nature are discussed, especially herbology, the use of plants as medicines. You can learn much from watching the cycles of nature and the daily motion of the sun and the moon. *Staying Healthy with the Seasons* has many suggestions on how to incorporate this information into your life.

With the massive increase in chronic disease, we are becoming more aware of the imbalances in our everyday habits which stress our systems and lead to many symptoms and illnesses. Such lifestyle imbalances as dietary abuse; environmental and food pollutants; inadequate exercise, causing waste buildup; and chronic mental and emotional stresses, affect our daily health and have been linked to chronic diseases like diabetes, high blood pressure, heart/vascular disease, and even cancer. Many of these imbalances are discussed in this book. If they can be corrected early, it is possible that the chronic problems aforementioned may be prevented.

This book is a timely statement for all who suffer from occasional acute problems and for those already dealing with chronic diseases. Illness is not necessary! Daily attunement *is!*

Enjoy yourself!

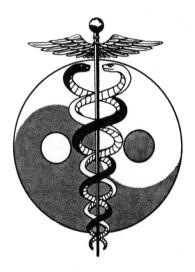

Ten

Carrying body and soul and embracing the one,
Can you avoid separation?
Attending fully and becoming supple,
Can you be as a newborn babe?
Washing and cleansing the primal vision,
Can you be without stain?
Loving all men and ruling the country,
Can you be without cleverness?
Opening and closing the gates of heaven,
Can you play the role of woman?
Understanding and being open to all things,
Are you able to do nothing?
Giving birth and nourishing,
Bearing yet not possessing,
Working yet not taking credit,
Leading yet not dominating,
This is the Primal Virtue.

from the TAO TE CHING
Lao Tsu,
translation by Gia-Fu Feng.

Before You Begin. . .

STAYING HEALTHY WITH THE SEASONS doesn't have to be read cover to cover. You might start by doing the Health Report Card, and then read the section for the specific season which you are in, then try the Basics section which lays the groundwork, and continue on from there. Then you could go back and use the book through the year, reading about each new season as you go, and preparing for changes.

But for those who are interested in this book as a health study, I suggest that you read *Staying Healthy* completely through, making notes and picking areas of interest for review, then check through again, using charts and tables which may not have been totally clear at first, and which may need some patience and focus. You might wish to go to other books for aid on particular topics, and incorporate all this with your own notes and ideas. You will find a bibliography in the back of this book.

Above all, I hope you enjoy this work and find that it helps you to "bridge the gap of credible realities" and achieve a growing awareness and responsibility for your own well-being, using the many gifts which nature has provided.

Basics

A Bit of Philosophy

An important change is happening in our view of health. It stems from a dissatisfaction with the ways in which we deal with our illnesses and the superficial approaches usually taken to remedy them. We realize that we need to experience health. We are seeking to go beyond the band-aid, the finger in the dike, and the treatment of various symptoms as complete approaches to any problem. Deeper and more substantial communication must take place with our environments and within ourselves. I believe that any illness invites us to take a moment, sift through the many levels of our existence, and ask for understanding and be open to needed changes. When illness arises, stop, look, and listen!

Basically, when we experience dis-ease, there is a message trying to come to us which we are not receiving. This message will persist until we see it. We can either be open to it, avoid it, or even hate it. Any resistance can create a conflict or struggle, and this is the nature and degree of our illness. We are all aware that most aspects of our lives are not constant. Our life force may persist, yet our experiences, feelings, and activities change regularly. Outside, nature does her dance. She is our teacher. She has her patterns, yet we cannot count on or expect anything for sure. Ancient wisdom states that, "Change is the only truth in the universe," or, "There is nothing permanent except change." If change is all we expect, we're stepping into the driver's seat.

We cannot limit ourselves to treating a disease. We must go further and deeper to understand the process and causative factors and then do progressive work on these. Many times the apparent disease is really a process in which the body is attempting to make itself better.

The weather varies continually, yet there are other natural patterns which affect us, like day and night, new moon and full moon, and the seasons—all important to our lives. Internally, we also have cycles known as "biologic clocks." These clocks regulate our daily hormone levels and metabolism, the menstrual cycles, the rapidity and degree of childhood growth, and the onset of adolescence and menopause. Other internal cycles are reflected in our emotional, mental, and physical energies as well as more subtle ones which influence our creativity, compassion, appreciation of beauty, our self-awareness, and our spiritual awareness.

There is indeed as much to be aware of within ourselves as there is outside us. This is an important key to health. We must take the time to check our inner senses regularly to feel what is happening and incorporate this new information into our lives. When we stop growing, or we resist our changes, we are liable to get sick. We must maintain our bodies in a relaxed and open state to keep energy flowing—inside to out, and outside to in—how else can we really experience life?

Body tension is created by resistance to energy flow, and illness often follows this accumulated tension. In order to stop impending changes, we must maintain this resistance/tension. Many times in our lives when we feel something is being asked of us, or we ask something of ourselves, we may experience feelings of fear, anger, or anxiety, and this may become the resistance to our change or growth. Can we stop nature? We can slow her by intervention, like damming a river, or cementing a cliff upon which ocean waves are crashing, but eventually nature has her way—the message comes forth —"Change!"

Brain(s): Hemispheres

Much attention and research has been given recently to the functioning of the two sides of the brain—the left and right hemispheres. The left hemisphere is considered "dominant" and controls the right side of the body. (In a percentage of left-handed people, the opposite may be true: the right hemisphere is dominant.) The dominant hemisphere is your active self, relating to the form and activity of your outside world and is concerned with time. This holds your waking consciousness, your linear thought—your rational side, which houses the speech center.

The right hemisphere, called "subdominant," is linked to the unconscious for most people. Some rarely experience this side in a waking state. It is your "other half." This is your nature side, your instincts, your artistic, creative source, and is not necessarily rational. No time, only space exists in this realm, as in the child's mind; it gives rise to your dreams and fantasies. Here it all exists as one.

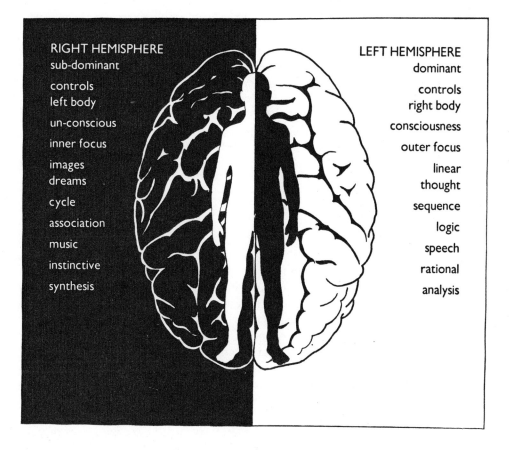

RIGHT HEMISPHERE
sub-dominant

controls
left body

un-consious

inner focus

images
dreams

cycle

association

music

instinctive

synthesis

LEFT HEMISPHERE
dominant

controls
right body

consciousness

outer focus

linear
thought

sequence

logic

speech

rational

analysis

Brain Waves

The mind's activities can be described as brain wave patterns, measuring the amount of electrical activity in different parts of the brain. There are four basic rhythms: *Beta, Alpha, Theta,* and *Delta. Beta* is from 12–24 cycles per second (cps) and relates to the active word or number thinking, when you may be making plans or solving a problem. The *Alpha* rhythm,

8–12 cps, is the so-called resting state, the background hum when the brain is recharging—nothing is going on; you are not thinking. The *Theta* state is 4–8 cps and related to the visual and dream states, thinking with pictures, wandering through space, through past pleasures and future excitements. Relaxing and picturing a scene in your mind will produce this rhythm. The *Delta* rhythm is slowest and relates to deep sleep. It is from 0–4 cps.

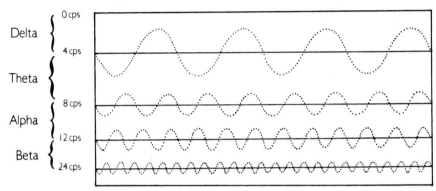

Dreaming

While dreaming, there are predominately two rhythms: *Theta*, visual imagery; and *Beta*, the processing of this vision. *Alpha* rhythm will show up at the quiet areas of the brain but all rhythms occur during sleep. The part of sleep where you obtain your deepest rest and where you dream, is characterized by a "rapid eye movement" (REM), with a *Beta* rhythm. The active eye motions apparently occur as you watch your dreams happen. In experiments, when people are deprived of their dreams (REM sleep) for several days, their behavior can range from very irritable to psychotic. Because this dream sleep is so crucial to physical, mental, and emotional health, you should work to recognize your dreams and bring them to consciousness, and even to record these experiences of your unconscious self.

Dreams may be premonitions of your own or another's future, communications with your spiritual being, expressions or realizations of deep feelings, or just releases of excess mind-stuff and apparent nonsense. Whatever, they are intriguing, and you can learn to interpret your dreams so they have real meaning in your life.

In nighttime sleep and daytime relaxation, when your awareness is hovering somewhere between conscious rational thought and the anything-goes, timeless unconscious, you may experience these visions of your deeper self—the balancing or passing of energy from one side to the other (i.e., right brain to left) and from below to above (unconscious to conscious). In the center is your awareness.

Regular dreaming awareness suggests that you are close to the balance between your inner and outer worlds. If you lead an active life, are very busy all day and under some stress, have a hard time relaxing, and rarely dream, you are likely out of balance on the linear "real" world side. It makes it a little harder to recharge your batteries daily or alleviate tension. Often then, you must get sick to get the proper rest needed. Conversely, if you should have waking visions, hear voices, and consequently cannot take care of your earthly needs, you would be out of balance toward the inner, dream world and it would also be hard to manifest any dreams. When a person's life becomes totally controlled either by the material world or by the visionary world, he or she may experience faster aging, greater physical-mental stress, or confusion, sometimes labeled as neurotic or psychotic. Since these difficulties are not very well understood and often cause fear in others, many who suffer them have trouble in active society.

You cannot look at or interpret dreams on a totally rational basis. Often, things seem strange, or apparently make no sense, or go to extremes to make a point. Violent expression in dreams may just be the releasing of a bit of suppressed feelings; even the death of a friend or relative in a dream might mean merely that you are in a process of releasing yourself from an emotional attachment to that person, rather than wishing earthly physical death. Dreams may help you realize your conflicts or hidden emotions. You may meet and converse with friends or "spirit guides" in your dreams and actually receive some clear answers to questions or problems you have.

We can all benefit by being as close to our dreams as we are to our work—they hopefully reflect each other. Much guidance, inspiration, and realization ("Eureka!") may occur from watching and incorporating your dreams into your life. Keep a pad and pen near your bed and just record a few words or a line or two if you awaken from a sleeping vision. When you arise in the morning, those few words may restimulate the entire dream and you can record it fully. You may be surprised when you look back at these dreams a few months later and realize that some actually became experiences in your life. Enjoy walking the tight rope of inner and outer space.

Mind-Body Harmony: Health or Illness

To achieve the greatest awareness, your two aspects, right and left, mind and body, must stay in regular communication. By listening within, being aware of your body processes, your cycles, your true nature, you will keep growing and maintain your health. If you become too active, too absorbed in something you've created, too attached or too resistant to letting go of it, then your inner nature, which is concerned with your self growth as part of the evolution of our species, will try to communicate to your consciousness. If your consciousness is too busy, or your active mind cannot, relax, and new, vital information cannot get through, it will find alternative ways to communicate. This expression will in turn move from subtle to gross levels: for example, from dreams, visions, and life experiences to the mental and emotional levels, and then to the physical. The active side of yourself will finally have to acknowledge the needs of the physical body, and, when the body doesn't work correctly, attend to its repair.

The desire of your inner nature to change against the resistance of the body is the conflict which creates disease. What is manifested on the grosser levels is a specific symptom or illness which relates particularly to the message that it is trying to communicate, and this message is contained within the illness. The understanding and message is released when this dis-ease is unwound. If you suppress this information with tensions, or with drugs to mask the symptom(s), then this energy will become harder to clear as it goes deeper into the body. If you continue to relate to the process of illness with an attitude of battle, messages for potential growth will get suppressed, and soon you will have increasingly tense or painful places in your body, and more serious or chronic illnesses developing. Your only choice for continuing well-being is to stay open and integrate these experiences as they occur. Such an "expressive" rather than "suppressive" approach to illness will give you better health in the long run. Illness can be a vehicle to enhance your personal communication and facilitate your evolution.

"Unused evolutionary energy is the matrix of pain (and/or transformation)."

JACOB ATABET
Michael Murphy

Body/brain mechanics are not too dissimilar to a computer, which has certain data, a receiving place for new information, and an active place where the program can be carried out. No new information can be programmed until the computer is at rest. The same is true in the brain. While the mind is actively thinking, it cannot receive new internal or external information. To receive, it must stop a moment and listen.

You must help create the chance for this flow back and forth to happen. If you just move out of the way and allow it, the body will balance itself. This is one secret to maintaining health and preventing illness. You occasionally must stop and reevaluate, then go forward. Daily, relax the mind and body. Listen. Look within. Have no fear, all changes are positive; it's just your attitude that can get in the way.

Can we learn to use illness as our ally instead of our opponent? This is very important.

This inner self is the instinctive, intuitive self which sees and feels things before they happen. To stay in tune with your deepest self is to stay in tune with nature. Nature also seems to reflect the consciousness of humans, and gives messages accordingly. "Natural disasters," like personal crises, help with awareness and reevaluation. It seems that crisis as well as vanity are the two main concerns that stimulate people to take positive action toward self-improvement.

Each of us is truly our primary doctor with nature as our guide. We have all the healing knowledge we need within our very beings. Learning to make contact with the healing ability within and using this knowledge in our daily life is the route to better and better health and well-being.

Let us enjoy this experience we call life!

Allopathic Medicine

Allopathic, or Western, medicine is the current form of medical practice in America. *Allopathic* means "treating sickness oppositely," i.e., giving a medicine for a symptom or illness which may counteract it by causing an opposite reaction. Examples of this would be treating diarrhea with a drug which slows the intestines, treating asthma with a medicine which dilates the bronchial tubes, or treating congested sinuses with a drug which contracts and dries the sinus membranes.

Western medicine has made great advances scientifically and technologically, yet it has some weaknesses and limitations. It has a good ability to probe deeply into the human

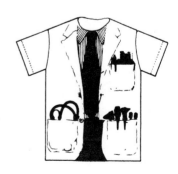

body in order to diagnose its anatomical and physiological conditions with its laboratory and x-ray testing. It has, confusingly to the lay person, developed its own language encompassing thousands of processes and symptom-complexes to give us the names of a multitude of maladies. To paraphrase William Osler, famous physician of the early 20th century, "One wonders if the pathologist with all his detailed and flowery descriptions of our body illnesses, may not, in fact, be creating these very diseases."

Western medicine has made great breakthroughs in acute care treatment with its technological advances in emergency care, its antibiotic development for infectious diseases, and its surgical intervention for trauma and advanced illness. However, the two-edged swords of its powerful medicines, anaesthesia and surgery, and invasive detailed diagnostic measures may relate to the large increase in the incidence of chronic diseases in our culture. These days most medicines are laboratory-made synthetic chemicals with side effects which can create symptoms and illness as well as treat them, and many of the diagnostic tests include irradiation and injecting various chemicals and dyes into the body. I hypothesize that some of the tests and the medical/surgical treatment for disease have a suppressive effect on the illness causing the energy of the symptom(s) to disappear by going deeper into the body rather than actually eliminating it. Suppressive kind of treatment may even lead to later crises or chronic disease, whereas expressive treatment seeks to eliminate the conflict of disease by reestablishing complete mind-body communication.

There is a purpose for all available medical models, and allopathic or Westen medicine certainly has an important place. However, with more of a focus on education and prevention, with a dietary sense and awareness of environmental and stress issues, a clearer and healthier human being will have greater disease resistance and less need for antibiotics and potentially harmful diagnostic and treatment measures.

Homeopathy

In contrast to allopathic medicine, homeopathic medicine applies the idea of treating "like with like." Termed the "Law of Similars", it means treating someone's condition with a substance that would cause the same symptom(s) in a healthy person. The effect of this is to undermine the illness and cause its elimination from the body—called the "initial aggravation." This corresponds to a worsening of symptoms, a brief return of difficulties of past illnesses before one begins to improve. This idea is common to many natural healing modalities.

Homeopathy is a medical science which uses elemental substances, both minerals and salts, triturated (diluted) to minute concentrations, and made into little pills (with a lactose, or milk sugar, base), to stimulate the clearing of symptom-complexes from the body, primarily by strengthening the individual's natural response. Homeopathy also seeks to use only a single remedy.

The law of cure describes that an effective treatment will cause symptoms to leave the person in a specific pattern: from the inside (deep) to the outside (superficial), from more important to less important organs, from the top to the bottom of the body, and from the most recent to the oldest symptoms.

In general, homeopathy uses minute doses, frequently administered over a longer period of time than those of allopathic drug therapy. It also takes into consideration the personality and the emotional and mental condition of the individual. However, as in all modalities, its effectiveness lies in the skill of the practitioner and the faith and commitment of the patient.

Law of Cure

Healing moves symptoms from:
1 inside to outside
2 top to bottom
3 more important to less important organs
4 most recent to oldest symptoms

Prevention

What is prevention? Really it is common sense and moderation in all things. This even includes moderation in moderation, meaning that occasionally we need to go to our limits. However, going to an extreme too often can lead to acute illness or chronic imbalance.

Prevention has two aspects. The first I call "avoidance." This means not doing certain things because they seem to us to be unhealthy or to cause certain problems. This includes such things as smoking, heavy alcohol or drug use, and overeating, but avoidance may be very individual as well. For some it may mean avoiding certain foods such as refined sugar and salt, fried foods, or animal products. For others, it may be not living in a big city, or not working in office buildings under excessive electricity and fluorescent lights, or even avoiding automobiles.

"An ounce of prevention is worth a pound of cure."
Benjamin Franklin

Healing Work
You can work on yourself only when you are ill and you'll usually return to the place where you started. Or you can work on your growing health and not become ill. The willpower and discipline for proper care of nourishment, exercise, and self-awareness is not easy, but nothing that pays off is. If you work toward health, the dividends will be higher day to day and you will feel better and positively love life.

The second aspect of prevention I call "positive action." This means doing something now, or on a regular basis, to keep us healthy or to prevent some specific malady from occurring. It includes all forms of exercise, from physical exertion with sweating, which helps stimulate the cardio-respiratory system and build strength and endurance, to the more passive and stretching/breathing forms which reduce physical, mental, and emotional stress and stimulate and balance the functioning of the internal organs.

Other "positive actions" include developing optimistic attitudes toward life, as well as all forms of relaxation and meditation, increasing inner awareness and relieving that stressed feeling. Really, all things that you enjoy or that nourish you will have this therapeutic effect. They may include such things as a walk in the woods, talking with the family, reading a good book, taking a sauna or hot tub, massage therapies, or deep breathing.

Nutritionally, there are also things which I consider "positive action." These include occasional rest from foods, and enhancing elimination, called "cleansing," by drinking solely liquids like fruit and vegetable juices and broths. This aids in weight loss, allows rest to the digestive system and internal organs, promotes rejuvenation, and improves vitality. My experience shows me that this process prevents illness, gives one a youthful appearance and vigor, and may affect longevity. Certain diets also have helpful effects and finding your own best diet is part of your prevention program.

How I incorporate prevention into my practice of medicine comes from the traditional Chinese doctors. I see people at the start or end of each season to evaluate their state and discuss any changes needed to adapt to the coming season; then I do an acupuncture treatment which will realign them with the new time. This concept of continual adaptation is the basis of this book. In old China, the doctors were only paid to keep people well. When their patients became ill, they had to take care of them free of charge. That's some kind of insurance policy!

Prevention really involves self-education and self-awareness, being in touch with what you need. You can then understand your patterns and use your knowledge to stay healthy. The following three systems—Nutrition, Herbology, and traditional Chinese medicine—all incorporate the subtleties of keeping the body finely tuned. They help you to understand the relationship between man and nature, and provide you with therapeutic models which can help strengthen and balance your body and sustain your good health.

Nutrition

Food is the body's fuel, and the quality and quantity you use makes the energy on which your wonderful body machine runs. What you eat helps create who you are, what you do, and how you feel. Use the appropriate fuel for vitality, good performance, and longevity.

Nutrition is of widespread concern and controversy, and varies widely throughout the world and indeed, within each culture. The climate, your activity and metabolism all affect your dietary needs.

Foods have certain components—carbohydrates, fats, proteins, vitamins, minerals—which are used in specific body functions; but foods also have general actions within the body. For example, fruits and vegetables help toward good elimination. Called the body "cleansers," they keep the body clean and light. Bread and cheese may be more binding and heat-producing, but they also create congestion and add weight.

The body "builders" are mostly the protein foods, for example, all the flesh foods, dairy products, nuts, beans, and seeds, avocados, mushrooms, tofu, and whole grains. These foods may also have a congesting effect, especially the meats and dairy products. Other "congestors" are breads, cakes, cookies, candies, soft drinks, sugar products, flour, noodles, potatoes, corn, and all processed and chemical foods. Too much congesting food can block the body functions and lead to stagnation and illness. Oils, butter, and margarine (unheated and in minimal doses) act as "lubricators," aiding the mucous membranes, intestinal elimination, and the joints, tendons, and ligaments.

You must all find your own optimum diets, but a good beginning might include mainly cleansing fruits and vegetables and whole grains, with some builders according to your activity and the climate in which you live. Only a little of the lubricating and congesting foods is required, and an avoidance of chemical additives in foods, as well as overeating. Chemi-

Seven to Heaven

1 Eat only when you are hungry.

2 Take a moment before eating to relax and breathe deeply—prepare for your nourishment.

3 Eat slowly and chew well.

4 Eat only as much as you need.

5 After eating, relax a while, then do some light movement, like walking, to help digest, assimilate, and circulate nutrients.

6 Do not eat for two hours before bedtime.

7 Eat a balanced diet.

FOOD ANALYSIS   VITAMINS   MINERALS

all figures based on 100 gm. of foods listed:	CALORIES	CARBOHYDRATE	PROTEIN	TOTAL FAT	FIBER	A	C	E	Comb. B 1,2,5,6 Niacin, Folic Ac. B	Comb. B12 & Biotin B	SODIUM	POTASSIUM	PHOSPHORUS	CALCIUM	IRON
		gm.	gm.	gm.	gm.	i.u.	mg.	mg.	mg.	mcg.	mg.	mg.	mg.	mg.	mg.
FRUIT APPLE, raw	53	13	.17	t	1.0	83	10	.74	.3	1.0	1.1	100	9.5	6.7	.5
ORANGE, raw	45	11	.9	.2	.5	190	50	.24	.8	1.0	1.0	18	20	40	.4
BANANA, raw	85	22	1.1	.2	.5	180	10	.4	1.7	4.0	1.3	366	26	8	.6
CARROT, raw	42	9.7	1.1	.2	1.0	11,000	8	.45	1.2	3.0	47	341	36	37	.7
VEG. SPINACH, raw	25	4.3	3.2	.36	0.5	8,028	50	2.25	1.7	7.0	70	466	39	90	2.7
POTATO, baked in skin	90	20	2.5	.1	.6	t	20	—	1.6	—	3	490	60	90	.7
ALFALFA SPROUTS	41	—	5.1	.6	1.7	—	16	—	2.0	—	—	—	—	28	1.4
SEA. NORI	—	44	35	.7	4.7	11,000	10	—	7.0	—	600	—	510	260	12
VEG. KELP	—	—	6	1.0	6.7	—	20	—	11.5	—	3,000	5270	238	1092	3.7
NUT ALMOND, raw	606	20	18.5	55	2.7	—	t	15	5.6	18.0	4	784	511	237	4.7
PEANUT, raw	600	21	27	50	2.7	t	—	6.7	14.0	35	5	721	418	74	2.3
BEAN KIDNEY BEAN, ckd.	121	22	8.5	.5	1.6	5.5	—	—	.9	—	3.3	349	143	39	2.4
SOYABEAN, ckd.	130	11	11	5.7	1.6	28	—	—	.9	—	2.2	540	178	73	2.7
GRAIN OATMEAL, rolled, ckd.	55	10	2.0	1.0	.2	—	—	—	.3	—	.3	61	57	9	.6
SEEDS SUNFLOWER, dried, hulled	580	21	25	49	39	50	—	—	11	—	40	952	867	124	7.4
SESAME, dried, hulled	582	18	19	53	24	30	—	—	6.9	—	60	925	822	1100	10.5
DAIRY MILK	65	4.7	3.5	3.4	—	143	.9	.12	.5	2.5	49	144	96	119	.04
EGGS	142	.8	11.4	11.3	—	1,040	—	1.0	2.4	22	108	114	180	48	2.0
FISH HALIBUT, ckd.	100	—	21	1.1	—	444	t	—	10.0	3.5	54	593	213	13	.7
FOWL CHICKEN, breast, ckd.	75	—	17	4	—	60	2.5	—	8.0	.5	84	362	170	8.6	.9
MEAT BEEF, reg., ground	270	—	18	21	—	35	—	—	6.6	1.2	—	237	157	10	2.7
MISC. SUGAR, white granulated	385	99	—	—	—	—	—	—	—	—	1	3	—	.1	—
HUMAN MILK	69	6.9	.9	4.5	—	247	4.9	.23	.5	.5	16.5	53	13.2	33	.03
YEAST, Brewers	283	39	39	1.0	—	t	—	—	60	800	121	1894	1753	210	17.3

cals in the diet and overeating both stress the liver, digestive system, heart, and kidneys as the body is either unfamiliar with the chemicals or has too much to handle. Start reading labels and be responsible for what you put into your only body.

With a clean system and good assimilation, you can extract from foods all that your body needs for daily use. However, if you get a deficiency from poor foods or eating habits, or cannot digest or assimilate well, you may need vitamin or mineral supplementation to replenish your lost nutrition.

The misuse of foods and other substances we call "foods" is a main factor in the formation of many acute and chronic ailments. The "common cold" and "flu" are primarily signals that the body needs to clean and rest itself. Overindulgence in foods, improper intestinal elimination, and the intake of more toxins (unusable materials) than the liver or the kidneys can detoxify result in a buildup in the tissues and organs. This must be regularly balanced by the abused body in bouts of elimination which we know as "illnesses." Intoxicants like nicotine, alcohol, sugar and caffeine, as well as the sprays and chemicals used to grow and prepare foods, affect individual organ functions and weaken the whole system.

On a long-term basis, certain diets contribute to specific ailments. For example, animal fats and cholesterol probably relate to heart and vascular disease and refined sugar and obesity are connected to adult diabetes. The initial studies of the relationship between diet and cancer indicate that certain cancers are associated with specific dietary imbalances, like that of breast cancer's association with an affluent diet rich in animal fats and colon/rectum cancer's similar relationship to high-meat diets which are also low in fiber foods. However, we can safely say that one's attitude toward one's life, along with lifestyle and amount of stress, are very important to what one's body can handle before it becomes ill.

Diet increases stress or reduces it. It can create disease or help heal illness. It even plays a role in changing the body's size and shape. To understand the nature of food and to learn how to create a health-full nutritional program for yourself is indeed important.

Proper nutrition does not relate only to the mouth organ. All of your sense organs have their food which helps to nourish and comfort them. The eyes eat light and color; ears live on

Food Labels

It is very important to you (and those you feed) that you learn to read and understand food product labels. Besides the common additions of salt and sugar to many packaged foods, there are natural and artificial flavorings, stabilizers, preservatives and many harmless and harmful chemical additives used in the processing of food. You, the consumer, can easily gain label knowledge if you need it. It is vital to your long-term health not to pollute your body regularly with chemical non-foods, and to enjoy more fresh and flavorful foods.

"We can create a healthy body by using fine foods and eliminating toxins."
RAYS OF DAWN
Thurmon Fleet

sound; the nose thrives on smells; the heart absorbs feelings; the skin, sunlight; and all of your cells and organs breathe and need good clean air to live.

So much of your health is in your own hands, learn to nourish yourself!

Herbology

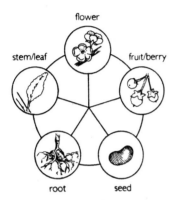

flower

stem/leaf   fruit/berry

root   seed

Herbology, an ancient and universal healing art and really the original American medicine, is the study of plants with medicinal properties and their actions and uses. While herbs have some effect in the acute or advanced stage of an illness, this is not their primary use. In fact, the stronger chemical drugs may be more appropriate for treatment in these situations. But herbs are very helpful as first-aid remedies for cuts, bruises, sprains, and so on. However, their main work is to achieve a more subtle effect on the whole body—cleansing, building, and balancing over a longer period of time.

Specific herbs have specific properties. Herbs can act as diuretics (clear excess water from the body), diaphoretics (cause sweating), expectorants (expel mucus from the pulmonary system), alteratives (alter bad conditions to good), or as demulcent-emollients (soothe and soften tissues), as well as tonics, cleansers, etc. (See Herb Glossary.) Most herbs have multiple effects.

An exemplary use for herbs is as a tonic or strengthening agent. Many herbs have a tonic effect on specific organs or systems in the body. For example, comfrey root is a tonic for the lungs and mucous linings, dandelion root for the liver, red raspberry leaves for the uterus, and nettle tonifies the kidneys.

To achieve a long-term tonic effect, you would use an herb daily in small to moderate doses over a period of weeks, or months, as a tea or encapsulated powder. A tonic dose might be one tablespoon of herb per cup of water prepared as a tea, once or twice daily, or two "00" capsules of powdered herb twice daily. Herbal formulas can be used in an individual to balance certain systemic and/or specific imbalances.

Taking the herb lavender (*Lavandula vera*) as an example reveals the multiple ways herbs can be used. First, the *beauty* of the growing plants and spectrum of colored flowers is nourishing to the eyes. Lavender's purple flowers are quite aesthetic. The *aromatic quality* of the plant has a wonderful effect especially on our subtle spirit and temperament. There is a whole subclass of herbology known as "aroma therapy." Lavender flowers and their perfume have been used for headaches and nausea, in preparation for childbirth, and in helping expel the afterbirth, as well as for freshly scenting closets and drawers. The third main use of herbs is for their *internal* effect. Teas from lavender flowers or leaves have been used to prevent fainting, allay nausea, and for vomiting or stomach troubles. Another common use of herbs has been as seasonings in cooking. Lavender is one seasoning herb. Others are basil, oregano, thyme, rosemary, and marjoram.

Another herb that grows throughout the United States and has multiple external and internal uses is plantain (*Plantago major*). There are two varieties: broad leaf and long, or lancet, leaf. Both plants are usable. Plantain has much traditional folklore surrounding it, and is also known as "Indian buckwheat" and "nature's band-aid." The tall shoots that grow from the plant contain the seed and flower. When broken apart, the individual seed containers look like tiny buckwheat kernels. The Indians gathered the young shoots and broke them up, mashed them with water, then took the flourlike paste, and made little patties, baked them in the sun, and ate them.

The therapeutic properties of plantain are as an alterative, diuretic, antiseptic, astringent, styptic, and vulnerary. As nature's band-aid, it is particularly healing for external sores, ulcers, burns, and stings from insects or plants. Crush or lightly chew some fresh green leaf, apply this to the wound, cover with several whole leaves, then wrap and tie the long shoot to hold the bandage in place.

Plantain's history also shows its use for hemorrhoids, eczema, boils and carbuncles, vaginal discharge and all sorts of women's complaints, diarrhea, and bladder or kidney problems. Used daily it is said to promote fertility. The chewed root may be helpful for toothache. It is a good herb to know.

There is a tendency for novices to overuse certain herbs that have an apparently good effect. Goldenseal root goes into this category. It is a powerful tonic especially for the digestive system and mucous membranes, being particularly helpful in eye, nose, and teeth or gum problems. However, in large doses or when used for too long, goldenseal can adversely affect the liver, gall bladder and other internal organs.

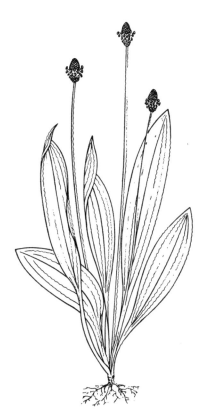

Plantain
Plantago major

Herbology, thus, can be seen as a sensitive system of healing, especially when used by someone aware of its subtleties. This knowledge may be acquired by taking the time and observing one's interaction with these medicinal plants. Herbs can also be used along with other health systems.

Chinese Medicine

The traditional Chinese system of medicine, thousands of years old, exists still because of its beauty and simplicity. It ties together man/woman and nature and the harmonious communication between them gives their mutual health. The age-old concept of seasonal changes affecting human growth and well-being was rooted and developed in ancient China.

The life force, or *chi*, is present in the two primary forces, *yang* and *yin*. These are dualities or polarities reflecting opposite states in continual interchange. *Yang* is pure energy corresponding to heaven; *yin* is substance and represents earth. *Yang*, the "male," active, light principle, is that force which wishes to expand into everything; *yin*, the "female," receptive, dark principle is the force that wants to contract into nothingness. The interaction of these two forces is what determines the very nature of the universe; their relationship is manifested as the five essential elements which make up all things.

The *Five Element Theory* is a primary relationship in the Chinese system. It relates all energy and substance to one of the elements—Fire, Earth, Metal (or Air), Water, and Wood. Each is associated with one of the directions of the compass and one of the seasons, with the element Earth being the center direction, relating to the season of late or Indian summer.

The process of the Five Elements runs through birth, growth, maturation, harvest, and storage. In daily life, we see idea, action, manifestation, communication, and reflection back to re-creation. Each element has a color, two body organs, a tissue it governs, and many other associations.

At the end of each seasonal section which follows there is a chart showing the attributes of that particular element. The relationships and associations of the complete Five-Element Cycle are summarized in a folded chart on the last page of the book. It might be helpful to refer to it now, as you become acquainted with the basic principles of Chinese medicine.

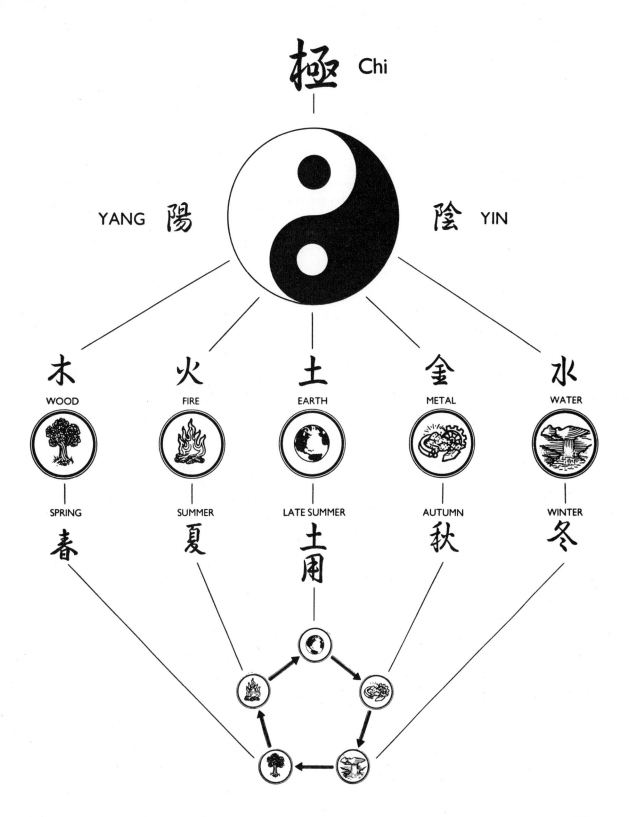

極 Chi

YANG 陽　　　　　陰 YIN

木　　　火　　　土　　　金　　　水
WOOD　　FIRE　　EARTH　　METAL　　WATER

SPRING　　SUMMER　　LATE SUMMER　　AUTUMN　　WINTER
春　　　夏　　　土用　　　秋　　　冬

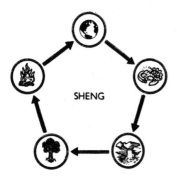

SHENG

The Creation Cycle

There are two major kinds of relationships within the Five Elements. The first is the "Creation," or "Sheng" cycle, also called the "Mother-Son Law." One element gives birth to the next and nourishes it by a flow of energy. For instance, Wood gives rise to Fire which creates Earth. Therefore, Fire is considered the son of Wood, and also the mother of Earth. The full cycle runs: Wood creates Fire creates Earth creates Metal creates Water creates Wood (see chart).

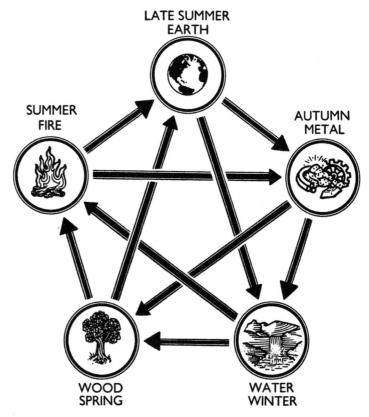

LATE SUMMER
EARTH

SUMMER
FIRE

AUTUMN
METAL

WOOD
SPRING

WATER
WINTER

The other relationship among the elements is called the "Ko," or "Destruction," cycle. This is really the "control" cycle since it represents the process by which the elements check and balance one another. However, if any get too weak, or too strong, they can attack another or be injured. Wood will injure Earth (root penetration), Fire destroys Metal (by melting it to liquid), Earth controls Water (dams), Metal attacks Wood (with an ax), and Water injures Fire (puts it out).

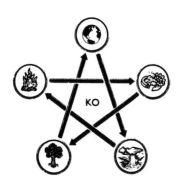

KO

The Destruction Cycle

According to Chinese legend, the Five Elements arrived from the different compass directions accompanied by the climactic factors, and continued on to create the world and the human body. In *Healing Ourselves,* Naboru Muramoto states: "The *east* creates the *wind;* wind creates *wood.* The forces of *spring* create wind in heaven and wood upon the Earth. They create the *liver* organ and the *muscles* within the body . . . and the *eyes,* and the *green* color, and the *sour* flavor . . . the emotion *anger,* and the ability to make a *shouting* sound."

Illness is classified as either *yang*—hot, in excess, and near the surface; or *yin*—cold, deficient and deep. The causes of illness are external and internal, termed the "devils," or "harms." External causes mainly include the climates, which, when extreme, penetrate a weak organism and injure a specific organ. The "perverse" climates which can cause illness are wind, heat, humidity (dampness), dryness, and cold. External factors also include bacteria and other infectious agents, poisons and pollution, and traumatic injuries. The internal causes of illness are emotions like excess joy or sadness, anger, depression, obsessiveness, worry, grief, and fear. Other internal causes are tension, overexertion, dietary maladjustment, excess sexual activity, excess mucus, blood clotting, and heredity. Each "harm" may affect a specific organ. Cold and damp can injure the lungs; hot and dry affects the heart; emotionally suppressed anger can injure the liver; while excess fear can endanger the kidneys. Each organ has a specific climate and emotion which can weaken it and leave it most vulnerable. An injured organ or weak system is of course more susceptible to illness.

By learning to adapt to external changes while you recognize and clear your inner experience, you learn to maintain health. When you are out of balance, you are more sensitive to change and susceptible to illness. At times of great energy shifts, such as the coming of a new season, the increased stress can make you more vulnerable to sickness. Thus, during these periods you may need greater awareness and care.

Nature influences man and man influences medicine. As nature changes, eventually so must medical practice. It always has. Thus, present practice in China reflects the strong influence of Western medicine, along with traditional Chinese herbology and acupuncture.

"When speaking of one day, the morning is governed by Spring, afternoon by Summer, evening by Fall, and night by Winter. The Spring energy gives birth; the Summer produces maturity, the Fall is the time for gathering in, and the Winter is a time for storage."

NEI CHING*

"Fire had been Shen Nung's (2820–2647 B.C.) patron element, for which he was also called the Red Emperor. His successor, who is said to have reigned from about 2697 to 2595 B.C., called earth his patron element. Thus, in deference to the earth's color, he was named Huang-ti, the Yellow Emperor."

CHINESE FOLK MEDICINE

*All quotes marked NEI CHING are from *The Nei Ching: The Yellow Emperor's Classic of Internal Medicine,* interpreted by Ilza Veith.

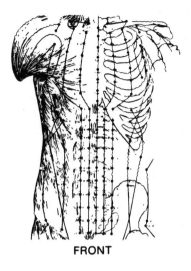

FRONT

The acupuncture system describes the circulation of energy in the body through a series of channels called *meridians,* in which the life force, *chi,* flows. Just as with the blood, lymph, and nervous systems, there must be an open flow to maintain health. Your environment and everything you think and feel affects the flow of this energy. When the *chi* flow is upset for a period of time, then physical symptoms may manifest. When the flow is open, and the organs are strong and functioning, there is balance, and all is well.

Every 24 hours, the *chi* flows through the entire body and the twelve meridians in a specific pattern, such that for each two-hour period one organ is dominant. This flow can be mapped out anatomically along the meridians. As an example, the peak energy for the lungs occurs between 3 and 5 A.M. If this organ/meridian has excessive energy, it may become most apparent during this time. Twelve hours from the peak time is considered the low energy point of the day for that organ, that is, 3–5 P.M. for the lungs. If symptoms occur from a weak or deficient organ, they may appear during the low energy period. If you observe the anatomy of the meridians, you can follow the continual flow of one meridian to the next throughout the day.

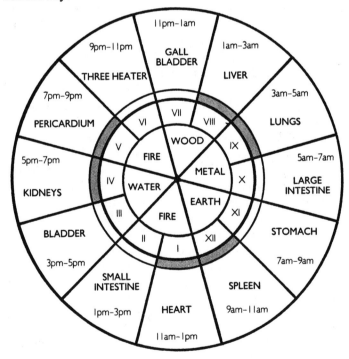

This introduction to traditional Chinese medicine has presented a simple overview of the concepts of the ancient Oriental theory of the human body, nature, and life, and how they are all connected. It takes patience and practice to get a real grasp of it; then you begin to see an evolved system which offers a penetrating view of illness and health.

In the following pages, we will go through the year season by seasons. Each season is represented by one of the five elements and the systems introduced in the "Basics" are explored more fully. Read these chapters to learn and re-learn more about yourself and your relationship to your environment, and to experience this relationship in a new light. This new knowledge will help you to prevent illness and stay healthy through the seasons.

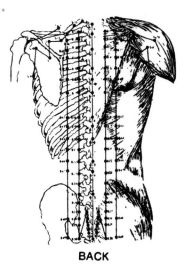

BACK

"Do not mistake acquirement of mere knowledge for power. Like food, these things must be digested and assimilated to become life or force.

Learning is not wisdom; knowledge is not necessarily vital energy. The student who has to cram through a school or a college course, who has made himself merely a receptacle for the teacher's thoughts and ideas, is not educated; he has not gained much. He is a reservoir, not a fountain. One retains, the other gives forth. Unless his knowledge is converted into wisdom, into faculty, it will become stagnant like still water."

from LEAVES OF GOLD
J. E. Dinger

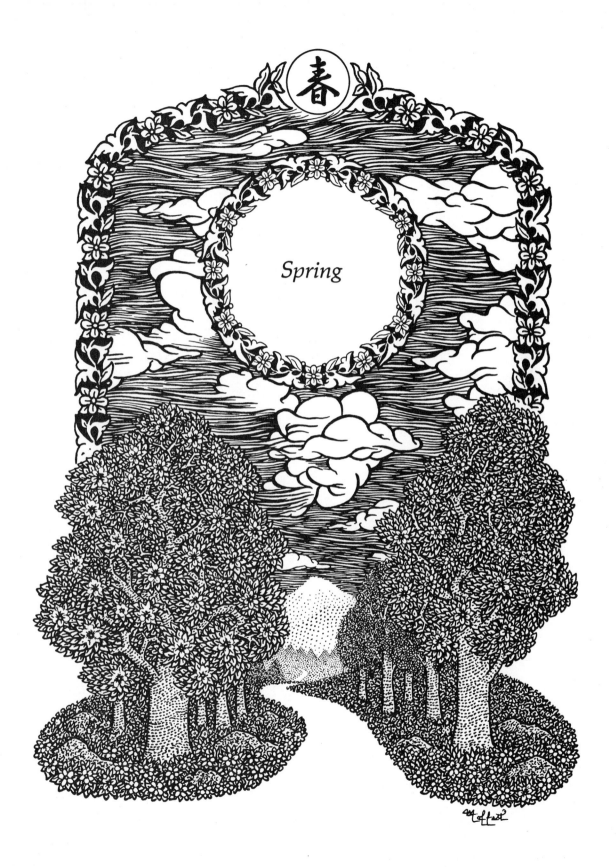

春

Spring

Spring Cleaning

HELLO. Oh, hello in there! Wake up! Spring is here. It's time to cheer, and shine like the sun. Come out and play; dance your dance. This is nature's birthing season—the time of creation and development. All is restored with life at the beginning of spring. That which is found within us in winter surfaces and wants to come forth in the full bloom of spring to be later nourished by the summer sun and bring the fruits of autumn.

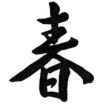

The beginning of spring is March 21st, the time of the spring equinox, when day equals night. For the next six months daylight, the sun and yang principle, will be dominating our lives. You may now feel a new spark and power, and be filled with inspiration and energy to act upon your ideas.

This is a good time to take a look at your life and make a new plan. What do you want to clear out as the past in your environment and within yourself—and what do you wish to see happen this year? This can be a *new start*. Take a little time to write a new health/life plan, including goals for how you wish to feel and what you would like to do and see happen. Let those dreams blossom.

Spring is the greening season. It is the time for planting. After the rain and snow of winter, the seeds begin to sprout from the depths of the soil, trees bud, and nature awakens in her green, flowering beauty. New growth in our lives, relationships, and work is stimulated now as well. We and nature will flourish this season.

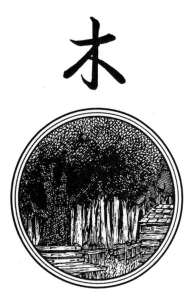

Wood Element

In the Chinese system of the Five Elements, the spring season is correlated with the element Wood, which governs the gall bladder and liver. The Wood element refers to living, growing entities: trees, plants, and the human body. They grow simultaneously out and upward, down and inward. The development of the root structure, as well as its early nourishment by sun, air, water, and soil, provide the strength and growth to the organism. Each entity has its individual requirements in these areas.

The Wood element refers to the growing structures; the roots, trunk, and limbs for the trees and plants; the spine, limbs, and joints in the human. A Wood imbalance can result in spinal problems, poor flexibility, or a weak-rootedness of an individual. In the Chinese system, arthritis is viewed as a Wood problem.

The color associated with this element is the predominant one of spring—the green of young plants. Someone who either is very attracted to the green color or really dislikes it is showing that the Wood element is possibly imbalanced. If this is the case, a greenish hue may be apparent on the skin of the face, especially on the cheeks and around the eyes.

The nature of spring and the Wood element is described as beginning or birth. Mentally, this corresponds to the "idea." The Wood element creates our mental clarity and our ability to focus, plan, and to make decisions. A Wood imbalance may be manifested in poor judgment, planning, and organization, with an inability to make decisions; or a very strong, over-developed Wood element may result in excessive mentality; for example, a person trying to organize everything and everyone. This person may have a hard time relaxing and may be prone to headaches and neck and back tensions.

The direction associated with the Wood element is east—the beginning or creation of the day as the sun rises in the east. This element rules the morning and a healthy Wood element gives one the capacity to arise energized for the day. A sluggish liver will make a slow morning riser.

The climate for the spring and Wood element is characterized by *wind*, which clears the old and brings the fresh, new air, like the transition from winter to spring. Wind nourishes the Wood. However, too much wind may be harmful. So in spring, if the Wood (or liver) is weakened or injured by over-exposure to extreme winds, one may get symptoms associated with an unbalanced Wood element, like poor resistance to illness or allergic sensitivities with its many symptoms, such as sinus or skin problems or irritated, watery eyes.

The eyes are the sense organ for the liver and Wood element, thus sight is the sense, and tears are the fluid. The *Yellow Emperor's Classic of Internal Medicine*, says, ". . . the eyes are connected with the liver, therefore they (and the vision) are strengthened when the liver receives blood." Problems of the eyes, vision, or tearing mechanism are often related to a Wood imbalance.

Each element has, along with its sense organ, a specific "indicator," and both may be observed to get an idea of the health/balance of that element. The nails, especially the toenails, are the Wood element's indicator, so you may check both the eye tissue and the nails for the state of health of the liver and Wood element in the body. Of course, this is only one way of checking the balance of the elements.

"The liver is ruler over the spring. It is the root of life's ultimate action; its condition is revealed in the fingernails and toenails as well as in the muscles."

CHINESE FOLK MEDICINE

The Wood element is associated with the sour flavor, and the *Nei Ching* says, "the liver craves the sour flavor." Some sour foods will nourish the liver; too much can cause problems. A person who craves sour or vinegary foods or who has a real distaste for them may be revealing a Wood imbalance.

The emotion of anger and the sound of shouting are related to the Wood element. If you feel these inside, you may wish to express them in a safe way. Suppressed anger may injure the liver and gall bladder. In general, a balance of energy allows you to experience and express all the emotions. Held-in emotions of any kind may breed disease.

". . . the liver has the functions of a military leader who excels in his strategic planning; the gall bladder occupies the position of an important and upright official who excels through his decisions and judgments. . ."

NEI CHING

The tissues governed by the Wood element are the muscles, ligaments, and tendons, those parts which hold us together and give us both strength and flexibility. If these areas are problematic, there may be an imbalance, weakness or congestion in the Wood element, either in the liver itself or in its energy channel, the "meridian." Muscle fatigue and weakness are two possible difficulties.

The Wood element gives the ability or capacity for control. If one who has a Wood imbalance is met with a challenge or request for change, he or she may respond by trying to control, either his behavior or the situation. The Wood element is also said to give the spiritual faculty to life; the liver is the home of the soul. This element gives us the inspiration and desire for life. If it is weak, we may lack the enthusiasm and spark to live. Remember, in the spring, all living things are restored.

Liver and Gall Bladder

The organs for the spring season, and the element Wood, are the liver and gall bladder. They carry out essential body functions, particularly the digestion and processing of many substances we take into our bodies.

The liver is the body's largest internal organ and is located in the right upper abdomen. It conforms to the under surface of the diaphragm (the breathing muscle which separates the chest from the abdomen). The lower liver edge can often be felt under the rib cage in the right half of the body.

While life itself depends on our lungs, heart, and circulation to bring oxygen, warmth, and nutrients to all cells in the body, the liver provides essential support to these processes, with more than a hundred known functions. We can't "live" without it, yet the liver has the amazing capacity to regenerate itself after surgery, injury, or illness.

The liver is the body's master laboratory. Essentially, it stores and distributes nourishment for the entire body, is involved in the formation and breakdown of blood, and filters toxins (unusable materials) from the blood. The liver (hepatic) cells make bile which aids in digestion, and stores the bile in the gall bladder to be used in the intestines for the breakdown (emulsification) of fats and for enhancing the small intestine's ability to absorb fatty acids.

Bile is a greenish, yellow liquid that contains water, bile salts, bilirubin, cholesterol, fatty acids, lecithin, and some inorganic salts. Bilirubin, the pigment in bile, is one of the end-products of hemoglobin, and thus one of the breakdown products of blood. When the liver, for a variety of reasons, cannot clear the bilirubin, the skin, eyes, and mucous membranes will pick up this green-yellow pigmentation. This most commonly suggests a liver problem, but may also result from excessive breakdown of blood cells.

The liver aids in the metabolism of carbohydrates, fats, and proteins, helping to keep the blood sugar level regulated by changing fats (lipids) and proteins (amino acids) into glucose (the simple sugar that all cells use) and back again for storage. Many of the enzymes which help catalyze the liver's own internal chemical reactions are produced by it. It also forms many gamma globulins and plasma proteins that assist in the body's defense system. The liver makes prothrombin which helps in blood clotting and two anticoagulants which prevent abnormal clotting: heparin and antithrombin. It can form vitamin A, and stores it along with other vitamins like D and B-complex. It also stores minerals such as copper, zinc, and iron.

The liver filters the blood of toxins and breaks them down for elimination. For example, it takes nitrogen wastes and turns them into urea which it sends to the kidneys for excretion. The liver can deactivate hormones like thyroid and the sex hormones, thus influencing the metabolism.

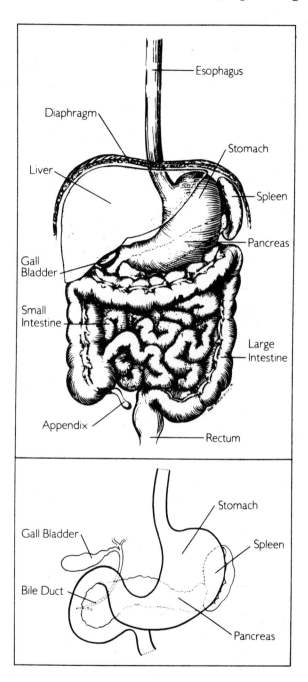

From the natural viewpoint, when the liver is overloaded, it is less able to detoxify the blood, and poisons remain, potentially leading to many acute and chronic problems which manifest themselves in each individual's weaker areas. Overeating can lead to an enlarged, overworked liver. Too much of any food, but especially alcohol, chemicals, drugs, fried oils and meats, can be toxic to the liver and gall bladder.

The gall bladder sits beneath and at the front edge of the central area of the liver. The gall bladder stores and secretes bile for digestion, especially for the breakdown of fats. It actually concentrates the bile by allowing absorption of water. Improper function may cause gas and cramping in the abdomen, most commonly in the right upper abdomen, as well as "referred" pains to the shoulders and the back between the shoulder blades.

The Chinese acupuncture system describes a sensitive flow of energy which is affected by the outer environment as well as by thoughts and feelings. Its continual flow creates health and harmony while its disruption or blockage can lead to symptoms and disease.

Facing you, please find an illustration of the meridians for the organs (gall bladder and liver) relating to the Spring. As you can see, backup of the gall bladder energy may manifest itself in physical and mental tension, especially in the shoulders and head, but also in the hips and thighs, areas connected with the gall bladder energy pathway. In fact, headaches, both tension and migraine types, are related to the gall bladder in the Chinese system.

Nutrition

With springtime, there is an opportunity to look at old patterns in your life with a new awareness. So, let's look at a most important energy source for you, your body's fuel—foods.

The way you eat is a significant part of a healthy diet. Taking a special moment to relax before eating prepares your body to receive the full nourishment of your meal. You should not eat when you are tense or upset, or in a stressful environment. Breathe deeply, chew well, eat only what you need, and take the time to digest your foods.

Liver and Gall Bladder Meridians

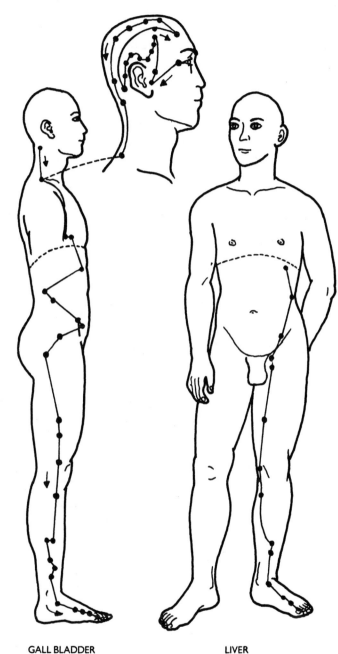

GALL BLADDER **LIVER**

Gall Bladder—44 points
The gall bladder meridian begins at the outer corner of the eye, runs over the top of the ear, then onto the head to the forehead and back over the head, onto the neck and shoulder, then to the front of the body, continues down the side of the torso to the hip; it then goes down the side of the thigh and calf, along the top of the foot and ends at the 4th toenail.

Liver—14 points
The liver meridian begins at the edge of the big toenail, goes along the top of the foot between the big and second toes, then runs along the inside of the calf and thigh and groin, onto the torso and ends just under the rib cage at the tip of the 9th rib.

Note: Meridians run on both sides of the body

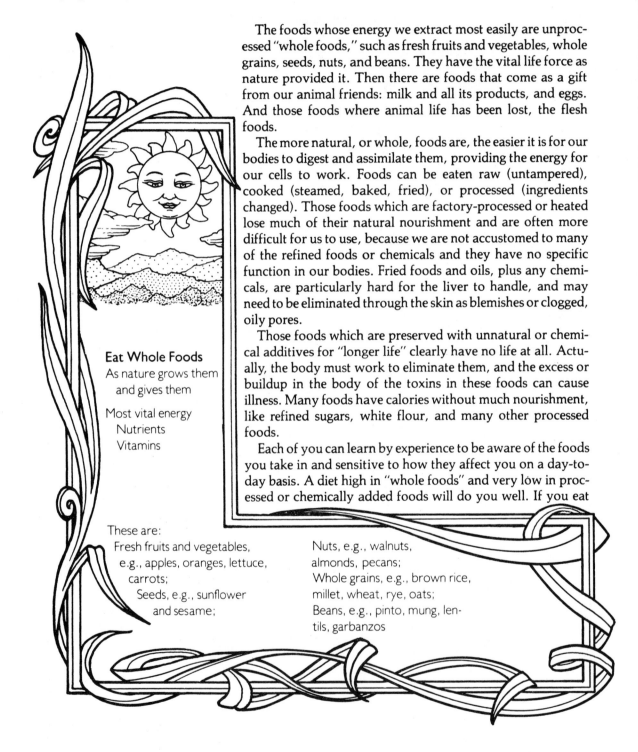

The foods whose energy we extract most easily are unprocessed "whole foods," such as fresh fruits and vegetables, whole grains, seeds, nuts, and beans. They have the vital life force as nature provided it. Then there are foods that come as a gift from our animal friends: milk and all its products, and eggs. And those foods where animal life has been lost, the flesh foods.

The more natural, or whole, foods are, the easier it is for our bodies to digest and assimilate them, providing the energy for our cells to work. Foods can be eaten raw (untampered), cooked (steamed, baked, fried), or processed (ingredients changed). Those foods which are factory-processed or heated lose much of their natural nourishment and are often more difficult for us to use, because we are not accustomed to many of the refined foods or chemicals and they have no specific function in our bodies. Fried foods and oils, plus any chemicals, are particularly hard for the liver to handle, and may need to be eliminated through the skin as blemishes or clogged, oily pores.

Those foods which are preserved with unnatural or chemical additives for "longer life" clearly have no life at all. Actually, the body must work to eliminate them, and the excess or buildup in the body of the toxins in these foods can cause illness. Many foods have calories without much nourishment, like refined sugars, white flour, and many other processed foods.

Each of you can learn by experience to be aware of the foods you take in and sensitive to how they affect you on a day-to-day basis. A diet high in "whole foods" and very low in processed or chemically added foods will do you well. If you eat

Eat Whole Foods

As nature grows them and gives them

Most vital energy
Nutrients
Vitamins

These are:
Fresh fruits and vegetables, e.g., apples, oranges, lettuce, carrots;
Seeds, e.g., sunflower and sesame;

Nuts, e.g., walnuts, almonds, pecans;
Whole grains, e.g., brown rice, millet, wheat, rye, oats;
Beans, e.g., pinto, mung, lentils, garbanzos

properly and balance your intake with regular elimination and exercise, you will experience optimum health.

Cleansing: An Important Part

Cleansing the body means to rid it of excess waste and dis-ease. This is done via resting from foods for a period of time and drinking juices of fruits and vegetables and/or water. This until recently overlooked process is important, even necessary, I believe, for good health and nutrition.

We can look at cleansing our bodies in the same way as we look at maintaining our automobiles. If we never checked them, retuned them, and cleaned or replaced clogged tubes, and continued to drive them, they would often break down. If they are evaluated and cared for regularly, they will run better, last longer, and not break down. So it is with our body, the most finely tuned machine on the planet. From its conception, it was designed to run on the pure, unpolluted, unprocessed fuel from the Mother Earth. Today with the varied and manufactured substances we eat, imbibe, and inhale, this cleansing is even more important to our vitality and health.

Most illnesses are a result of excess toxins (physical, mental, and emotional unusable materials) in the body. Healing is the elimination or cleansing of these toxins, and then achieving a balance of intake and output.

Fasting has been used throughout the history of mankind for a great many reasons. For example, Hippocrates employed nutrition and fasting in his practice—"Food is your best medicine." Fasting is actually an instinctive response (animals do it) to many illnesses, especially colds, flus, and intestinal problems. It has also been used in many cultures for physical rejuvenation and for enhancing vitality. Fasting has been employed for greater religious and spiritual awareness. It was often prescribed in the Eastern Indian culture, and the Essenes from the time of Christ used it to get rid of bodily decay, to cleanse their sins, and to realize God. Fasting is still used widely today for purposes of healing and individual clarity. I have found it a very useful tool.

The springtime seems to be the best time for major cleansing, drinking nourishing liquids, such as fruit and vegetable juices, for a period of five to ten days or longer. This differs from fasting, defined as water intake only. The second important time for cleansing is the autumn, to prepare for the next year's work—but we might do our cleanse early while the weather is still nice enough to go out for regular exercise and activity. The summer is an easy time to eat lightly with lots of fresh fruit and vegetables available, while the winter time is the hardest season to cleanse, especially in the colder climates where one needs more fuel to keep the body warm.

You may develop a schedule of liquids only one day per week or a three-day period monthly. It will indeed strengthen, lengthen, and lighten your life—preventing physical degeneration by eliminating toxic buildup in tissues and organs, allowing rest to the systems, and facilitating proper physiology.

Those who wish to do a long liquid cleanse, or who have acute or chronic illnesses, should best have medical supervision, though it is rare to have any difficulty other than willpower in a juice cleanse. On the other hand, a fast on water is a strong cleanse, often debilitating. I don't recommend this without close supervision.

Master Cleanser

**Stanley Burroughs'
Master Cleanser**

2 tablespoons fresh squeezed lemon or lime juice

1–2 tablespoons 100% maple syrup

1/10 teaspoon cayenne pepper

8 ounces spring water

Drink liberally (from 6–12 glasses/ day) throughout the day.

One cleanse that seems to work wonders, and is not very difficult for most people since it gives lots of energy while cleansing, is the Master Cleanser, better known as the "lemonade diet." It was the first cleanse I ever did, for ten days, and the experience changed my life.

The Master Cleanser formula is: 2 tablespoons of fresh squeezed lemon or lime juice; 1–2 tablespoons of pure, 100% maple syrup; and 1/10 teaspoon cayenne pepper, all mixed in eight ounces of water, preferably pure spring water. You can adjust this slightly to your taste, but most people find this a good balance of flavors—sweet, sour, and spicy.

Lemon is a perfect liver food and a great body cleanser. High in vitamin C, potassium, and other minerals, lemons are somewhat astringent, meaning that they contract and tighten tissues, which loosens up and clears the toxins from deep tissues and organs. My hypothesis is that lemons are an especially good aid to arthritis sufferers, cleansing the joint spaces. This very cleansing action can cause joint pains, which is why people with arthritis and their doctors may feel it is inappropriate but this irritation will pass, and the joints will feel improved.

The cayenne pepper helps clear the blood and eliminates toxins and mucus, as well as keeps the body warm. The maple syrup is wonderful energy (calories too), and it, along with honey, is a primary natural sugar. You may vary the calories and sweetness by using less maple syrup depending on the weight loss you desire, which can be up to two pounds a day, especially with lots of activity. Honey is not acceptable in this drink, as it is congesting in these doses.

Drink Master Cleanser as needed throughout the day, at least six glasses a day. One to two weeks is not too difficult or too long for this cleanse.

It is important for this cleanse to keep the intestines moving daily to clear toxins. Cold-pressed (unrefined and naturally pressed) olive oil, one tablespoon twice daily, is a good nutrient, liver tonic, and intestinal lubricant. For those who don't say "Ech!" a body-temperature water, or catnip tea enema will help clear the lower bowels. Catnip acts to relax the sphincter muscles and any spasms in the lower intestines. The tea is made by steeping a tablespoon or two of catnip herb in a quart of boiled water, cooling to body temperature, straining, then mixing with water into the enema bag.

"Internal salt water bathing," an oral rather than rectal intestinal cleansing, involves adding one quart of lukewarm water to two teaspoons (may vary slightly per individual) of *sea salt*, and drinking the whole quart first thing in the morning. Those people with high blood pressure or a tendency toward edema (swelling) should use caution with this method. However, this liquid should be in balance with the body fluids, so it usually passes right through the intestines without salt or water absorption. Your bowels should move a couple of times in the one to two hour period after drinking. You can do this every other morning while cleansing, adjusting the salt content if necessary. This means that if you try it and very little comes out, you may need to add a little more sea salt next time to the quart of water; or if a lot comes out and you get really thirsty, use a little less than two teaspoons the next time.

Drink a laxative tea in the morning and before bed. You can purchase an already mixed "laxative tea" at your health-food or herb store or make your own. Some herbs that you may use are licorice root and seeds like anise, fennel, or fenugreek. In a few cups of water, add a teaspoon of each herb, and simmer for 10–15 minutes, then let steep to drinking temperature. This is a mild laxative tea. Other herbs like cascara sagrada bark, senna leaves, or Oregon grape root have a stronger laxative effect, but may cause cramping in some people. Peppermint or

Internal Salt Water Bath Intestinal Cleanse

2 level teaspoons sea salt
1 quart lukewarm spring water

Drink whole quart first thing in the morning—do not eat until 1–2 hours after. Rest or exercise lightly, but stay near a bathroom.

other chlorophyll teas will also be an enjoyable treat on these days and will help neutralize body odors.

Bathing the skin and scrubbing it with a loofa sponge or skin brush is important for removing dead skin cells and washing off the toxins that have been eliminated through the skin. This is best done once or twice daily while cleansing, especially with good activity.

A new daily exercise is a great springtime idea, for example, jogging, tennis, jumprope, dancing, or swimming. These help build strength and endurance, and create a good cleansing sweat. Other more internal practices like yoga stretches, tai chi chuan (a subtle martial art/dance movement), or Feldenkrais exercises will help nourish you with your own vital energy, stretch those muscles, tendons, and ligaments, and put the "spring" into your joints.

You'll find that during cleansing you have lots of time and energy to get into your creativity as well as your normal day's work and responsibilities. As you continue, your eyes, vision, and other senses may get clearer along with your mind. Decision-making and the ability to follow through usually improve, and procrastination disappears. Take a couple of times daily to sit quietly, and focus on breathing freely, allowing the thinking mind to rest. Begin to see yourself as healthy and vibrant and active in the life you wish.

Breaking your fast, or cleanse, is the most important aspect of all. When are you ready? First, during your cleanse, especially in the first days, don't be alarmed by symptoms, such as a headache, or light-headedness, unless they persist or get worse. Even a mucus discharge from sinuses, chest, or intestines, or skin eruptions are not uncommon. Be prepared to rest if you feel weak, though it is not too usual. Also, make sure you drink enough lemonade, 6 to 12 glasses a day.

You may briefly experience your body's toxins, deeper tensions, or the symptoms of past and potential illness as you clear them out. You can check a couple of monitors. For example, during the cleanse your tongue may get coated white to yellow, then may clear again suggesting completion of the cleanse. Also be aware of your senses, mental clarity, emotional comfort, and ability to deal with what may have been at other times very frustrating situations. Observe your bowels and urinary systems to check your eliminating functions.

Basically, have faith and listen to your body and you will know intuitively when it's time to end your cleanse. Hunger may set in after some days of being absent, suggesting it is time to begin eating again, a little at a time. If weakness sets in after a period of days of strong, vibrant energy, it may be time to rest or to begin coming off the cleanse.

It is best to take *several days* getting back into solid foods, so your system doesn't overreact. After the Master Cleanser, try orange juice, fresh-squeezed and diluted half with water, for a day, then other juices like fresh apple or carrot-celery through the next few days. On the second day, a simple vegetable soup can be made; first drink the broth, then eat the vegetables later.

Progress slowly and eat lightly. When you begin eating raw foods again, don't overeat, and remember to chew well and make juice in your mouth. To quote from the "Anatomy Strip" song, "Chew-Chew Train" by Gary Guitar, regarding nutrition, "When you're hungry please remember, like a train go chew chew chew . . . What you eat and how you eat it makes you feel the way you do."

After the cleanse, you have a real opportunity to see and feel what each food in your diet does in your body. Certain foods may feel right for you—and others may cause reactions, like gas, general discomfort, a "stuffed" feeling, or a weakening of your energy.

Elimination Cleanse

You can do this checkup, if you wish, with a different kind of cleansing process, in which, if you have allergies, frequent colds, intestinal difficulties, or energy or mood swings, you can test to see what specific foods, or eating in general, have to do with your problem.

First, slowly, taking 7–10 days, eliminate various foods from your diet in steps: processed and chemical foods; drugs, including alcohol, nicotine, and caffeine; meats; dairy products; beans; nuts, seeds, and grains—then eat fresh fruits and vegetables only for 3 days, followed by 2 days of juices only (fresh squeezed when possible) 2 days of water only, and one day of juices. Now slowly, taking 7 days, introduce *one food at a time* back into your diet, giving 3 hours for each one, taking good notes on what it does to you and what you do with it. How do you feel?

Elimination Cleanse and Dietary Test

Start where you are and finish where you wish. It will take from 15–30 days.

For days when you are adding foods, test at least three different foods each day, and give yourself 3–4 hours to experience each one's effects. It is best if you eat a mono diet (one food at a time) for these days. However, if you need to include the previous day(s) category, you may, but still do your testing. Do a moderate dosage of any food you try. For example, eat 3 whole carrots, 4 oz. sunflower seeds, a bowl of brown rice, 4 oz. of cheese or a glass of milk at their appropriate times. And have a good time.

Day 1 Eat your normal diet.
2 Eliminate all chemicals from diet e.g., **food** additives, drugs (non-prescription), nicotine, alcohol, caffeine.
3 Eliminate all processed foods—refined sugar, white enriched flour and their products.
4 Eliminate meat products—any live or once living animal.
5 Eliminate dairy foods—all cow, goat, chicken products.
6 Eliminate nuts and beans.
7 Eliminate seeds.
8 ⎫ Eliminate grains, eating only fruits and
9 ⎬ vegetables. Eat fresh fruits and vegetables in
10 ⎭ raw, steamed, or juiced forms. (*3 days*)
11 ⎫ Fruit and vegetable juice and broth *only*. No cans—
12 ⎭ juices should be fresh or bottled, naturally squeezed. (*2 days*)
13 ⎫ Water only—spring or well—not tap water.
14 ⎭ These may be rest days. (*2 days*)
15 Fruit and vegetable juice again.
16 Fruit—one kind at a time (3–4 hours between kinds), one large or two small fruits.
17 Add vegetables.
18 Add grains.
19 Add seeds.
20 Add nuts and beans.
21 Add dairy foods.
22 ⎫ Add meat, only one kind per day
23 ⎬ and only if desired—you are
24 ⎭ now more sensitive. (*3 days*)
25 Add any processed foods—only if desired.
26 Add any chemicals or drugs—only if desired.

Begin with a few fruits, one at a time, eating an appropriate portion of each food. Then on subsequent days eat vegetables, grains, seeds, nuts, beans, dairy products, and finally meats— whatever you are comfortable eating, and see what happens. This whole process can take from 15 to 30 days (see chart) depending on where your diet begins and ends.

Take good notes, as they provide important feedback for you on how your body functions. It is also a nice healing experience. Check the correlation between your intake of foods and the elimination of feces. Also check your general senses and the eyes, tongue, skin color, general energy level, and whatever other monitors you feel are important.

During your cleanse it will be a good time to take an occasional sauna bath or hot tub to allow toxins to clear out through the skin. Remember the importance of exercise to keep everything moving. A good sweat helps body elimination and cleans the blood. The skin is a large organ which acts as the third kidney and third lung.

Body Therapy During Cleansing

This is especially a good time to experience different kinds of body therapy, for either general relaxation, clearing and/or restructuring. Body therapies may be on two levels, based on depth of work and on goals. On the one hand, massage may be geared toward a goal of relaxation and is usually a pleasant and sensual experience, done lightly with long strokes over the body's muscular system. Massage can also go deeper depending on the therapist and the focus, with particular areas isolated for working through painful, tense spots. We all have some of these.

There is also "therapeutic" massage, or body therapy, which works toward releasing tension and blocks in muscles, tendons, ligaments, and organs by affecting the energy patterns in the body. It often incorporates breathing exercises to help relieve stress. Mental relaxation, emotional awareness and expression, or psychological counseling, may also be important aspects of body work.

The goal of all of these is long-term relaxation by clearing energy channels and by releasing tensions, creating a greater body-mind-emotion harmony. Massage and body work therapies include Swedish and Esalen massage, Reflexology or Zone Therapy, Acupressure, Shiatsu, Polarity Therapy, Ortho-Bionomy, Feldenkrais, Alexander Technique, Postural Integration, and Rolfing, as well as Skeletal-Corrective procedures. But remember, just relaxing itself can be therapy.

Reflexology
Each part of the foot relates to a specific part of the body. Massage of these pressure points can be especially beneficial during cleansing.

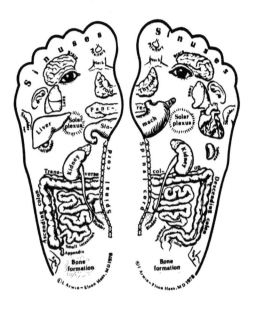

Here are a few more cleansing-related topics. First, a disadvantage for already trim individuals is the weight loss from extensive cleansing. Another potential problem is that cleansing does not totally discriminate against impurities, but other tissues, vitamins, minerals can be reduced as well. This is inconsequential for a healthy person involved in a cleanse of up to two weeks, but for a longer cleanse or for weak or ill individuals, cleansing may cause further depletion of certain body stores, besides some muscle reduction. For these people, taking vitamins and mineral supplements while cleansing may be a remedy, though this does interfere somewhat with the cleansing process. Another possibility which helps keep the body strong is to add a high-protein plant product, like *Spirulina plankton* or *Chlorella*, to the juices. A third solution is to do shorter cleanses, like one week, and alternate these with building diets including protein and rich vitamin/mineral foods.

A Cleansing Experience

Recently, on visiting family and friends after five years, I was made aware of how much I had changed, and of how many unhealthy family patterns had left me After returning home, I wrote in my journal about my experience of cleansing. . . .

At first the cleansing process didn't seem like what I wanted but I have to say, it is what I needed. Everyone has some limitations which they must get past just to begin. Well, this change wasn't easy for me, but it was so fulfilling, so worthwhile. There was a clearing of much of the excess I carried around—40–50 pounds of too much eating, of too much talking, of unexpressed feelings and desires—and I continued until I realized that to be really well, I had to hire myself to help out with a new and difficult job. I had to learn to balance my intake and output. I realized this, of course, after the experiences of greater intake and less output, in which I gained weight and then less intake and greater output, which is what has to happen to lose body mass. I began to see that this intake and output did not only concern food, but included mental activity, breathing, exercise, emotions, and creative expression. We can gain weight merely by not expressing what we feel.

With the Master Cleanser and other lightening and enlightening dietary aids, including support and firmness from dear friends, I totally changed my diet over a couple of years to enjoying the treats of Mother Nature—live and vital foods. I gave up eating my animal friends, as well as many other congesting foods such as sugar, processed foods, candy goodies, and all baked products, except for occasional whole grain products. And I switched to eating mainly the foods that could run this body most efficiently; good raw salads, juicy fruits, some steamed vegetables, whole nuts, seeds, and grains, seaweed (sea lettuce), tofu, and lots of sprouts that I grew myself from seeds and beans. It does work! I cleared out the old—congestion, fat, and diseases of the past, present, and future—that I carried around with me.

Then I had a series of colonic irrigations to cleanse the large intestine (colon) of the old stuck, unnatural, chemicalized, assembly-lined, barely digestible "food" and meats which I had packed away during my innocent youth and which were hiding in the corners of my tubes. This ancient form of water irrigation is still a powerful means of ridding the body of waste and disease. The colon may be our most distressed organ, and, I believe, the primary source for physical decay because of modern-day diets.

As my cleansing and healing moved along, I experienced a process of getting to know myself, of becoming aware of my inner being through several physical/psychological therapies with highly qualified practitioners, helping the opening and clearing of those held-in emotions. They felt good, especially when the sessions were over. Deep breathing, sweats, relaxation, and painful birthing of this self—these were all part of this finer tuning.

I began moving and stretching my body every day to open up and clear out old stuff inside muscles and joints, and breathing, rejoicing. Slow stretches, relaxation, breathing into the exercise, into the body part are all important.

I took time every month for three days of liquids only. I did this at new moon because at this time I felt more sensitive and tended to overeat, but it turns out that this is a Buddhist custom as well. This cleansing time helped to clean out and rest the intestines and the hard-working digestive system, and relax the entire body; this was when I really looked at the progress and the process. It was a time for me to catch up on the undones, to get clear, and to plan for the next cycle.

I found it easier, and very stimulating and important to express myself—both my feelings and my ideas. I became very busy in ever-growing, meaningful, productive work with people as their physician, helping them to feel better and to realize that their well-being was in their own hands.

A couple of other important concepts surfaced in my consciousness and my life. The first was the awareness of the planet Earth as an alive, whole being who gives to all of us and who is ill at this time, what with all that is being taken and the little given back. I believe that our individual bodies and lifestyles and how we care for ourselves and others have a direct effect on the planet.

I became aware of the use of every substance, where it came from and where it goes. Needless processing makes nature's resources less valuable to us. For instance, it is the quality of foods that establishes a good diet, not the quantity.

Recycling is also important, i.e., giving back for re-use anything that can be re-used. This includes returning paper, glass, cans, cardboard, to the companies who will re-use them, and giving all organic wastes, such as fruit and vegetable trimmings, back to the Earth. "Composting" these materials gives us fine soil for our gardens 6–12 months later.

Taking quiet time with myself regularly to check out how I really feel, listening to my inner self, helps me to become aware and sensitive to my whole being and what it is doing in this life. Ideas and projects and solutions may become clear at this time. The process of knowing myself and being closer to my feelings and expressing them is important to my health. Awareness of my needs enables me to give up more immediate pleasures and gratifications for long-range goals which really fit those needs.

I listen every day to nature and to my deeper self and ask that I do the work that I came here to do, with love. I thank God each day for this life, and pray that I only grow closer to the truth, to the Oneness of the Universe.

This is the story of my realization and my dedication to creating the healthiest body possible. Everyone may not need such intense or complex therapy, but while it takes work, it is worth it. What we put in really affects what comes forth.

Cleansing is a process which induces changes in your shape, your energy, your attitudes. After cleansing experiences, you are often sensitive to things you never noticed before. These may include people, environments, smells, foods, ideas, and more. Especially your taste for foods moves toward the natural flavors. This may seem a disadvantage to some, but if you are looking for growth, you will have to make certain changes to reach the goal towards which your body guides you.

This cleansing experience can also present problems for family units in which only one member enters this transformational process. Sometimes it may cause splits—one seeks to grow and change, the other is happy to be where he or she is. I explain this to people when they consult with me about cleansing programs, and encourage couples or families to cleanse together. A shared experience tends to bond people, and the support from loved ones is often the key to success.

I have used the support group and shared experience to create successful cleanse classes. For the past two years, in spring and autumn, I have guided group cleanses, ranging from 10 to 50 people, and most have made it through the 10 day experience. The feedback has been amazing and the individual effects very gratifying, creating needed weight loss, mental clarity, dietary changes, and enthusiasm for life. The secondary effects on family, friends, and the whole town were great also. People have said, "I feel great, extraordinary, better-than-ever;" "The experience changed my life;" "I'll never eat again; I feel so good." The editor of our local paper went through his first 10 day cleanse and he wrote:

FASTING IS FUN (AND RESTORATIVE)
I broke the fast I have been on (together with about 30 other people) after eight days instead of the recommended ten—my organs have all been flushed by the lemon juice, my blood purified by the cayenne, my palate titillated by the maple syrup—I recommend the fast to everyone—it gave me an enormous amount of energy and eliminated as well as accumulated toxins and excess proteins from my body, the word procrastination from my life by producing a clear DO IT NOW state. Greg H. said he was prepared to give an all out testimonial for the regimen, Michael L. said he had experienced a spiritual awakening and reminded us (at the meeting with director Elson Haas) that it was most unusual for so many people

to fast together for a week or so like this—for him it was quite wonderful.

For me too—it made me much more aware of what different foods do to my system particularly after the actual breaking as I began with the orange juice, moved through broth and then. . . ."

For those of you with allergies or frequent colds, these cleanses will relieve symptoms and also clear toxins and excess mucus from your body to make it a healthier one. You might also try nibbling daily a few local, edible flowers, in increasing amounts (just a taste at first, making sure you know which ones are edible), and brewing a tea from them as a desensitization process for allergies. It may be helpful to eat local in-season fruits and vegetables and to eliminate processed and chemical foods, as well as all sugars except small amounts of pure maple syrup, or local honey, from your diet. In fact, local honey seems to contain an anti-allergenic factor, being made from flower pollens.

Eat a good balance of moderate protein and the complex carbohydrate foods, with a high vitamin B content, such as the whole grains like brown rice, millet, wheat, or oats. High protein diets are falling out of fashion, they seem to be too rich for the human species on a long-term basis and may even be related to chronic degenerative diseases.

For allergy and cold problems, vitamin supplements, particularly a high-potency vitamin B complex, twice daily, along with vitamin C (1 gram, 5 times daily) should be helpful. If your problem appears at the same time every year, try cleansing for a couple of weeks before that time comes and see how it changes things.

Spring Diet

In your own cleansing experience, you may not wish to use only one specific juice; you can create your own program by drinking different fruit and vegetable juices each day. Some examples are citrus fruits, pear, apple, carrot, beet, celery, spinach, and parsley. You may need a juicer to make most of these. And remember, drink fruit and vegetable juices separately, as they don't combine well in the stomach. In general, more fresh fruits and vegetables are good in the spring diet as you lighten up from the heavier, more heat-producing diet of winter.

A refreshing drink, especially on a hot day or after exercise, is a "Spring Cooler" (summer, too!). Use a carbonated mineral water like Perrier or Calistoga, and mix in it some fresh orange, lemon, lime, or other juice. Sit down, relax, and drink this bubbling treat.

Greens

Greens have been a traditional part of the spring diet in most cultures. They are plentiful at this time of the year and their use has always been associated with freshening, cleansing, and building the body.

Some local green herbs around my neighborhood are chickweed, chicory, malvas, dandelion, and miner's lettuce. If you are not familiar with these plants, find someone who knows to show you around your area, and be sure to avoid taking plants from areas which might have pesticide residues or from busy roadsides. Take a long walk in the country or in local parks or hillsides to gather your greens. You can grow your own greens at home, like wheat grass or alfalfa sprouts, and juice or eat them, too.

The active part of all these plants, giving them their green color, is chlorophyll, which may be one of the strongest, true healing agents known to man. Chlorophyll closely resembles hematin, the substance that when combined with protein forms hemoglobin, the large molecule that carries oxygen in our blood. Whereas hemoglobin has an iron molecule at its center, chlorophyll has magnesium. This observation led to much research through the 1950s by many scientists looking for the effect of green plants and chlorophyll on anemia. Many felt that the animal body was capable of converting chlorophyll into hemoglobin, thus being a potential remedy for anemia. During the same time American surgeons found chlorophyll to have positive effects as a healing agent for wounds, peptic or gastric ulcers, and inflamed or ulcerated colons (by rectal implantation). How about another fresh look?

Green plants or chlorophyll absorb energy from the sun and water from the earth and make sugar, starch, and protein. Greens have a moderate amount of protein, from 10 to 20 percent, and many contain calcium, phosphorus plus the B vitamins, and vitamins, C, E, and A.

There is crude chlorophyll available on the market. However, growing your own greens and eating or juicing them will give you the fresh natural chlorophyll with all its positive effects.

Sprouting—Your Home Garden

Let springtime give you a new enthusiasm for life, and enough inner juice to turn that soil, plant those seeds, and begin your own garden. In the kitchen, too, growing and eating sprouted seeds, grains, and beans is truly creating and using your ultimate food. Almost any seed or bean will sprout, but I like to grow alfalfa and sunflower seeds, as well as spicy radish seeds, green peas, lentils, garbanzo, mung, and red aduki beans.

Put a handful of seeds or beans in a large glass jar and cover with about three times as much water. Use a cloth or piece of screen for the top for draining. Soak overnight or up to 24 hours, then drain and rinse them, and place the jar out of the sunlight on its side for two or three days, rinsing, draining, and shaking the sprouts gently twice daily. They like to stay moist, but not wet or too dry. Finally leave them in a spot where there is a mixture of indirect and direct sunlight for a day or two keeping them moist while they grow green with chlorophyll. Refrigerate in a covered container and use in salads, soups, or sandwiches.

In a quart (or larger) jar, place enough rinsed seeds or beans (unhulled) to cover the bottom. Fill the jar with water, cover, and let soak overnight or longer. Strain out the water and rinse with fresh water, leaving the seeds moist but not wet. Place the jar in a cool, dark spot and rinse the seeds twice a day for two to four days—don't let the seeds dry out.

After a couple of days, your seeds will sprout. Place the jar in a brighter spot, continue to rinse two or three times daily until your sprouts are green on the ends. Refrigerate and use freely.

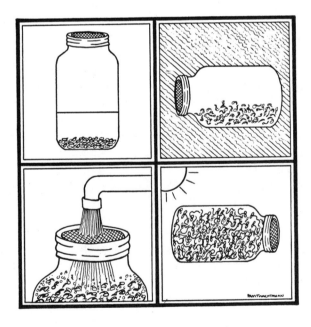

A simple enlivening salad is alfalfa and bean sprouts, tomatoes, and avocados, dressed with a little olive oil, lemon juice and seasoning. With a taste of honey added to the dressing, the children will love it too! And sprouts are highly nutritional and good protein foods, many being complete proteins. As most sprouts grow, their protein content increases; when they become green, chlorophyll and many vitamins are added and the protein ratio decreases.

Wheatgrass

The use of wheatgrass juice as a tonic and healing agent has risen in the last 10 years. The concentrated juice is rich in chlorophyll, vitamins, and minerals, and just drinking an ounce or two of it will give you a sense of its power.

Wheatgrass is the green tops of sprouted, hard red wheat. You can grow it in seed flats indoors. Over good seeding or potting soil, spread one layer of wheat, soak with water, and cover with a dark cloth or plastic. Leave for 2–3 days, checking only to make sure the seeds do not dry out. When the little roots reach into the soil, and the wheat begins to sprout, uncover, and keep it moist in a sunny window. Within a few days, you'll have 3–6 inch richly green wheatgrass, which you may use freely.

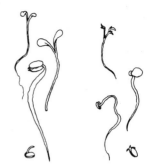

Sprouts
Most seeds, grains, peas, beans, even some nuts, will sprout. You can use alfalfa seeds alone, or mix several kinds together—lentils, garbanzos, mung, and/or aduki beans. Radish and fenugreek seeds are another nice combination.

Herbs

Several herbs are especially valuable for spring use. The first is sassafras bark (*Sassafras officinale*), a wonderful spring tonic with an enjoyable flavor. However, use this with caution, for safrole, the oil extract from sassafras, may have harmful effects in large doses.

Sassafras tea is known to purify the blood, and acts as an aromatic, stimulant, diaphoretic, and diuretic. It is also good for the skin and joints, and for the kidneys, bladder and chest. Its use may prevent colds and throat troubles. It's also a good stomach and bowel tonic and helps relieve gas. Used both internally and externally for skin eruptions, it has been helpful in easing poison oak and ivy, as well as rheumatism and arthritis.

Simmer one teaspoon of bark per cup for 10–15 minutes in a glass or stainless steel kettle, then pour into a pot over leafy

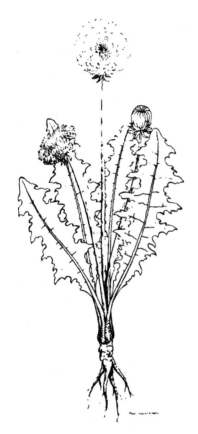

Dandelion
Taraxacum officinale

herbs like peppermint, nettle, or comfrey, and let steep for 15–20 minutes more. One cup of sassafras tea, taken daily for a few weeks, will help cleanse the whole system.

Dandelion (*Taraxacum officinale*) is another good springtime healer. The greens, very nourishing and high in vitamin A, are good in salads or used to make tea. The root is a blood and kidney cleanser, particularly a liver cleanser and tonic, as well as a diuretic. It can be used as a tea for jaundice and liver congestion resulting from liver-irritating drugs, and as a general cleansing stimulant for the liver. The roasted root is a nice coffee substitute, along with chicory root and roasted barley.

Roots in general should be simmered from 15–30 minutes, depending on their density and hardness, to extract their essence. For dandelion root, a medicinal dose is one tablespoon per cup, simmered about 20 minutes, then steeped another 15 minutes, three to four cups daily. In general, a tonifying dose for herbs is one tablespoon per cup once daily, taken over a month or longer.

Peppermint (*Mentha piperita*), a great herb for year round use, has always been a common household remedy, and grows prolifically in the garden. In spring, it has some special functions. Peppermint leaf tea is a good one to drink during cleanses as it freshens the breath and body odor, and is stimulating as well. Peppermint as a strongly made tea, or inhaled as an aromatic oil, is known to relieve headache and sinus pressure. It is also a nice cooling herb and iced peppermint tea is a good balance during the hot weather.

Peppermint herb is known to act as an aromatic, stimulant, antispasmodic, stomachic, and carminative. Its common use is for headaches, and to relieve nausea and vomiting, diarrhea, and stomach cramps. It has also been used for heart trouble, cholera and dysentery, convulsions, and muscle spasms. Applied externally it has been known to help headaches, rheumatism, and neuralgias.

Dr. Edward Shook in his *Elementary Treatise in Herbology,* suggests a tea made from equal portions of elder flowers and peppermint. He recommends this for colds and fevers and uses it for both adults and children.

Mix an ounce of each herb into a pot and pour 1½ pints of boiling water over them. Let steep for 15 to 20 minutes. Give a cup of hot tea to the patient who is in bed under lots of blankets with a hot water bottle under his or her feet. Sweating should begin by 30 minutes and continue through the night to help relieve the fever or cold. Adults can drink up to three cups of tea and children from one to two. They can drink water as needed through the night. In the morning, they should be sponged dry, put in a clean bed, and given a tall glass of fruit juice.

Many other fresh local herbs, greens, and flowers, surround us in the spring. Using locally grown, in-season herbs, fruits, and vegetables will help us to remain in harmony with Mother Nature.

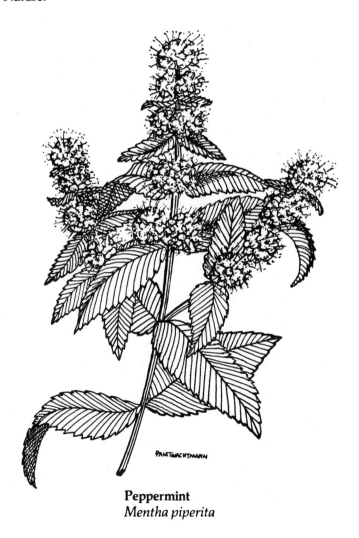

Peppermint
Mentha piperita

Summary

The seasons change; we change. When we move outside the laws of nature, or resist change, we encounter difficulty. If we learn to live within these laws we will know health as our friend.

Staying healthy through the spring season means keeping your Wood element—your liver and gall bladder—in the best possible shape, with new attention to your nutrition, exercise, self-awareness and self-expression. Spring is the season of beginning, creation. This is a special time to be open to the new, and the season to clear out the past which is ready to leave.

Nutritionally, it is a good time to fast, or to do a liquid cleanse, creating a clearer harmony between your inner and outer lives. Your diet will become lighter, with more raw foods—greens, sprouts, salads, fruits, nuts, seeds—some grains but fewer heavier foods like meats and dairy products, avoiding fried foods, chemical foods, and alcohol and other drugs.

Mental relaxation will allow you openness and peace of mind, while developing your ability to focus and to make clear decisions. Physical activity will help to clear and open the body and mind. Developing a regular exercise program is important now.

Making contact with your creative self is vital to spring harmony. Who are you inside? What do you need to express to feel free? You are continually creating your life; be aware of this, and dance and play the tune that you are!

As you can see, a lot is going on in the springtime of life. It is important to clear out the past to create spaces for the future to come into being *now*. If there is no room for it, the new energy will get all clogged up in the system. When spring arrives, remember, "elimination equals illumination."

Spring

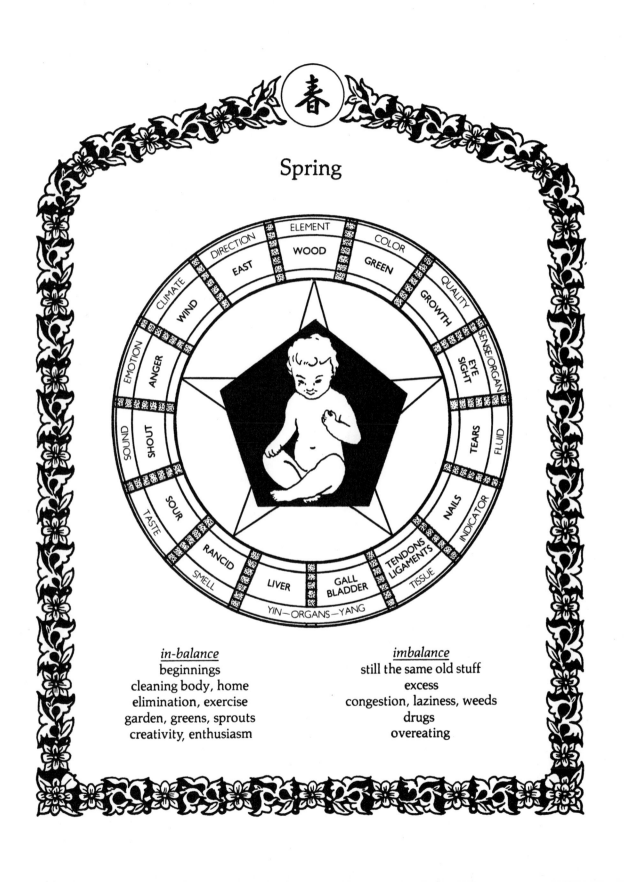

| DIRECTION | ELEMENT | COLOR |
| EAST | WOOD | GREEN |

CLIMATE — WIND · QUALITY — GROWTH · SENSE/ORGAN — EYE/SIGHT · EMOTION — ANGER · SOUND — SHOUT · FLUID — TEARS · TASTE — SOUR · INDICATOR — NAILS · SMELL — RANCID · TISSUE — TENDONS LIGAMENTS

YIN — ORGANS — YANG : LIVER · GALL BLADDER

in-balance
beginnings
cleaning body, home
elimination, exercise
garden, greens, sprouts
creativity, enthusiasm

imbalance
still the same old stuff
excess
congestion, laziness, weeds
drugs
overeating

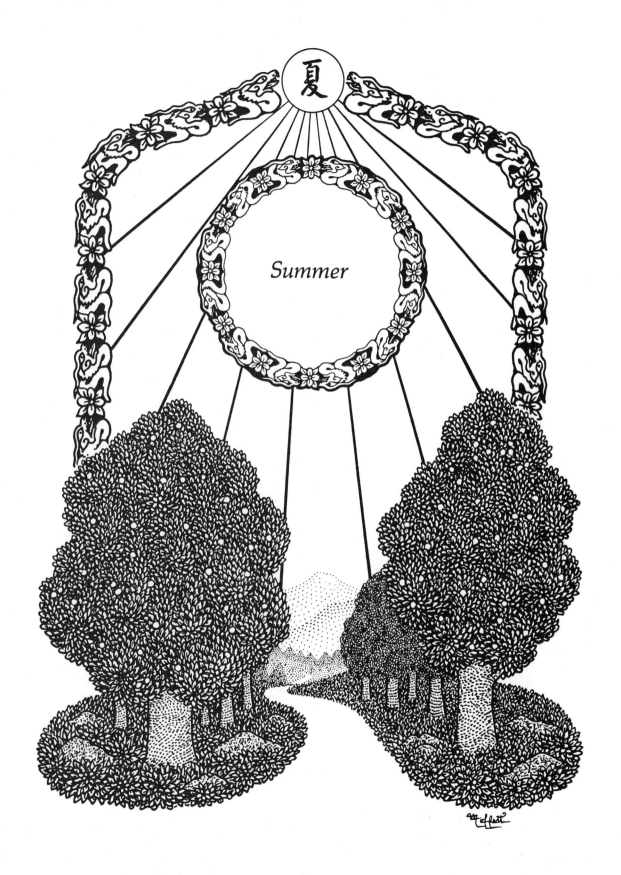

Summer Light

WE ENTER SUMMER on June 21st with the summer solstice, when the sun is at its northernmost position relative to earth. At the solstice, we have the longest daylight of the year. The sun is considered *yang* as it gives energy, causes action and outward movement, and creates the hot and dry climate. All this leads to the increased travel and working and playing in the beautiful sunshine. But this solstice day also marks the beginning of the cycle of growing darkness, or *yin*, which will peak six months later at the winter solstice.

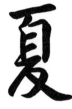

Summer is nature's season of growth and maturation. Flowers and fruits are all around us and our gardens are growing tall. We are equally maturing and growing, and this is the high point of outdoor exercise, sports, water recreation, and hikes in nature. We should make sure to get adequate recreation and lots of solar energy this season.

There are a lot of changes going on now. The Chinese health philosophy and its theory of the Five Elements give us a good awareness of such change, both in nature and in our bodies, which really mirror each other. Energy must stay in motion within us and in our life to continually nourish us and create harmony.

We must learn to flow as nature does, through the seasons. Tension happens when we resist this flow, and illness can occur when we resist our changes. Illness is usually a process which makes us more receptive, more open to change. This is often its value.

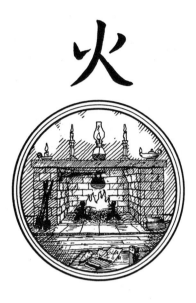

Fire Element

The element Fire, which, in the Chinese Five Element Theory characterizes summer, is seen as providing the energy governing the heart and small intestine. In addition, there are two other systems linked to the Fire element, so that it runs along four meridians (energy pathways), while each of the other elements has only two.

These extra two systems may be seen as physiological aspects of the Fire energy. The first is called the "circulation-sex," or the "pericardium," and this functions to protect the heart and to regulate the blood flow, heat, and nourishment throughout the body. The other system is termed the "three heater," "triple warmer," or "three burners," by the Chinese, and acts to maintain proper temperature and warmth.

The heart and small intestine, and the circulation-sex and three heater functions, are given symbolic roles. The actions of these four energies in the body give us an overall picture of how the organs all work together.

The heart has to do with the ability to rule, to understand and see clearly, and to serve compassionately. The small intestine functions to receive, digest, and assimilate nourishment. It sorts out and extracts the good from what we ingest. Professor Jack Worsley, noted teacher of acupuncture, describes this organ as the "separator of the pure from the impure."

The circulation-sex channel, also known as the "pericardium" or the "protector of the heart," regulates blood flow and sexual secretions. The *Nei Ching* says "The middle of the thorax (the part between the breasts) is like the official of the center who guides the subjects in their joys and pleasures."

The last organ function that the Chinese link to the Fire element is the three heaters. Its three burning surfaces are located at the mid-chest, where the upper burner relates to the heart and lungs; the solar plexus, where the middle burner relates to the stomach, spleen, gall bladder, liver, and small intestine; and the umbilical area, where the lower burner is associated with the large intestine, bladder, and kidneys. Their job is to produce heat and energy for the body through respiration, digestion, and elimination, respectively. Coolness over any of these three surfaces may suggest weakness in that specific function.

The two Fire functions, circulation and heating, are important to the overall harmony of the body.

"The burning spaces are like the officials who plan the construction of ditches and sluices, and they create waterways."

NEI CHING

Three Heater, Circulation-Sex (Pericardium) Meridians

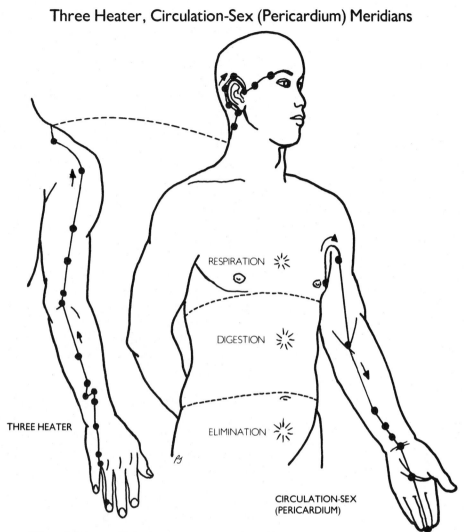

RESPIRATION

DIGESTION

ELIMINATION

THREE HEATER

CIRCULATION-SEX
(PERICARDIUM)

Three Heater—23 points
The three heater meridian begins by the nail of the fourth finger, goes up the back of the hand and over the wrist, runs along the middle of the outside surface of the forearm and arm, over the shoulder, up along the neck and around the ear. It ends at the point just lateral to the eyebrow.

Circulation-Sex—9 points
The circulation-sex meridian begins just lateral to the nipple, goes onto the arm and down the center of the palm surface of the arm and forearm, onto the hand and ends by the nail of the middle finger.

Note: Meridians run on both sides of the body

Fire is light and warmth, and its function in the body is to maintain heat, but also to give warmth to others. The Fire element gives enthusiasm, vitality, and energy. In the Chinese system, it also relates to the southern direction and to the color red. A strong attraction to or avoidance of red may represent an imbalance of this element.

This element is associated with the emotions of joy and sadness. Excessive joy or laughter, especially as inappropriate responses, are considered abnormal emotions, and these, as well as sadness, can create, or result from, an imbalance in the Fire element. Also, the ability to make the laughing sound comes from this element.

The flavor associated with the Fire element is bitter. Bitter foods and herbs are seen as strengthening to the heart and small intestine, though an excess of this flavor may injure them. We should learn to apply the maxim that if a little is good, a lot is not necessarily better; in fact, it may be harmful to us. Moderation characterizes the Chinese system, and practicing it is one of the keys to good health.

A balance of the five flavors in the diet—sweet, sour, spicy, bitter, and salty—keeps the body in harmony. The *Nei Ching* offers this wisdom:

If people pay attention to the five flavors and blend them well, their bones will remain straight, their muscles will remain tender and young, breath and blood will circulate freely, the pores will be in fine texture, and consequently breath and bones will be filled with the essence of life.

Fire is the most *yang* element, the most active, outward, and "masculine" energy. Fire is the Sun—energy, warmth, and vitality; and the sunlight is *yang*, noon being when *yang* energy is at its peak, and the heart's dominant time of the day is 11 A.M. to 1 P.M. Dawn and dusk have a balance between *yin* and *yang*, while midnight is most *yin*.

The Fire element relates to the energy of creativity, intuition, and motion; it is the action that carries out the "idea" from the Wood element. This action leads to the manifestation of the Earth element. Wood creates Fire which creates Earth. Fire people thrive on activity, on new ideas and ventures—on change.

Heart and Small Intestine Meridians

Heart—9 points
The heart meridian begins under the armpit, runs along the inner side of the palm surface of the arm and ends at the edge of the nail of the fifth finger.

Small Intestine—19 points
The small intestine meridian begins by the little fingernail. It runs up the side of the hand, along the forearm and behind the elbow, continues up the back of the arm and onto the shoulder above the scapula, onto the side of the neck, then the face, and ends in front of the ear.

SMALL
INTESTINE

HEART

Note: Meridians run on both sides of the body

Heart and Small Intestine

The two organs that correspond to the summer season and the Chinese Fire Element are the heart and small intestine. The heart, one of the organs most active in the summer season, is the regulator of the blood circulation, and the one to give attention to now. It is our own muscular four-chambered pump, which moves the blood as it carries the oxygen and other nutrients to the rest of the body. Its function is regulated by an intrinsic electrical system which keeps the steady beat, causing a contraction of the heart muscle via an electrical discharge.

The heart is finely sensitive to feedback mechanisms concerning our brain and muscle oxygen needs, which are communicated to the heart through the nervous system. Its rate and rhythm are also determined by our breathing and our mental and emotional states.

"The heart is like the minister of the monarch who excels through insight and understanding and fills the roles of 'sovereign ruler' from whom emanate directing influence and clear insight."

NEI CHING

This hard-working ruler of the body serves each cell's needs in pumping some 3,000 gallons of blood per day to the neighboring lungs, through which all blood must pass to obtain oxygen. Then the blood is returned to the heart, which pumps it out to the body, so all the parts can receive this nourishing breath of life.

Blood pressure is the force exerted by the blood inside the blood vessels. The determining factors of blood pressure are the force of the heart muscle contraction, the volume of blood, and the resistance of the blood vessels. The pressure changes as the heart beats. It is highest (systolic) when the heart pumps, and lowest (diastolic) when the heart is filling. The accepted measures for normal blood pressure are below 140/90, measured in millimeters of mercury (mmHg).

Average blood pressure is in the range 110-120/70-80 mmHg. Any pressure above 140 systolic or 90 diastolic for a period of time is considered high blood pressure, also called hypertension. This disease endangers the health of the heart and shortens one's life span. Factors that affect blood pressure levels are one's sex, age, weight, diet, activity, and the level of stress—physical, mental and emotional.

A treatment program for someone with mild to moderate high blood pressure, with a diastolic pressure up to 105, might include weight loss, a low-salt diet, regular exercise, and adequate rest. Also of vital importance is the relief of stress and avoidance of stressful situations, as well as avoiding cigarette smoking and drinking alcohol or caffeine.

This treatment may lower the diastolic blood pressure to 90 or below and then one will not need to use stronger drug therapy. However, the blood pressure should be checked monthly to make sure it does not rise again.

If the heart is weak or the blood vessel tone is low, then low blood pressure may exist. This most commonly occurs in the young, thin women who don't exercise. Low blood pressure can cause general weakness and lethargy, lightheadedness, slow mentality, and poor circulation. A generally good building diet will help this condition, but an active exercise program is the best remedy.

An indicator of the general state of the heart's health is the tongue, which in the Chinese system is the sense organ of the heart. In fact, the Fire element gives its energy to the function of speech.

The tongue should be moist and pink. If it is red, then the Fire or heart energy may be too strong, which could lead to an

Heart and Small Intestines

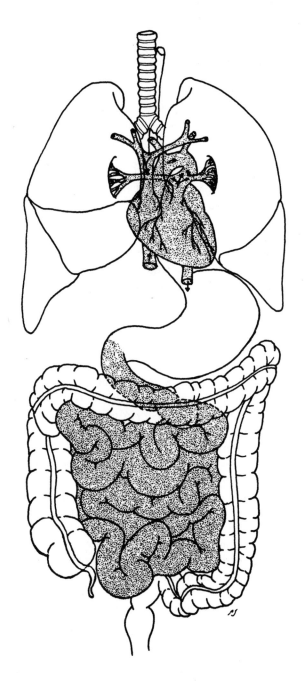

Heart—Source of Life
This central muscle pumps blood, carrying warmth, oxygen and nutrients throughout the body. It works closely with the lungs to gain oxygen and with the digestive system to obtain nutrients.

Small Intestine
This long organ with its large surface area works to digest foods and absorb their nutrients which it sends directly into the blood supply.

"The middle of the tongue is correlated with the stomach. The two sides of the tongue are correlated with the liver. The root of the tongue is correlated with the kidneys. The tip of the tongue is correlated with the heart. As may be expected, the coloring of the tongue is as relevant to the diagnosis as is the tongue's overall condition and fur."

CHINESE FOLK MEDICINE

inability to relax or slow down. If the tongue is pale, it may reflect weakness of the Fire element, as possible anemia. Anemia is a reduction of circulating red blood cells which may cause weakened capacity to carry oxygen and nutrients throughout the body. There are many causes but all affect the amount of circulating oxygen, and thus can create symptoms like lethargy, slowness in action and thought, and coldness, especially in the hands and feet.

A coated tongue relates more to diet and poor digestive functioning. If one smokes, a yellow-coated tongue is common.

To check the heart and circulatory functions, also observe the facial complexion color and body color, especially the fingertips and under the fingernails (red, pink, blue, white?). You might also check for any swelling, particularly in the ankles and shinbone areas. This could represent sluggish circulation, excess salt intake, or fluid overload.

The temperature of the hands and feet reveal the state of circulation as well as the general state of body relaxation. Warm hands and feet usually signify good heart and circulation function while colder hands and/or feet may mean weak circulation or increased tension. Nervousness and apprehension create constriction of the blood vessels in the wrists and ankles as part of the "flight or fight" response to deal with stress and potential danger. Relaxation is important for the heart and for keeping the rhythm of life.

The small intestine is the other Fire element organ. Its 23 foot length connects the stomach to the large intestine and is divided into three parts named the *duodenum*, the *jejunum*, and the *ileum*. This organ could also use care during the summer. The proper functioning of the small intestine is the key to our nourishment because the only nutrients we can actually use are those which we digest and assimilate through it.

The teeth and stomach work our food into a liquid state; then, with the help of the enzymes from the pancreas, bile from the liver and gall bladder, plus other substances, the small intestine transforms the foods we eat into usable components like glucose, fatty acids, and amino acids. These substances are absorbed into the bloodstream from the small intestine and transported to the liver, which either distributes them for immediate use or stores them in the form of glycogen for future use. Glycogen can be transformed back to glucose, fatty acids, or amino acids when needed by the body.

If the small intestine is clear and nutrients move at a reasonable rate, much can be absorbed, and the wastes carried on to the large intestine. However, if a great deal of mucus is present, coating the intestinal lining, or if the intestines move too fast (the feces are too loose), your body will receive very little nourishment from the food you eat.

If you occasionally rest the intestines by a few days or longer of juices, as described in the Spring section, and avoid a diet high in mucus-forming foods such as meats, dairy products, breads, and sugar products, you will keep your intestines in a state for proper digestion and assimilation.

"The small intestines are like the officials who are trusted with riches, and create changes of the physical substance."

NEI CHING

Fire-Water/Male-Female Relationship

When we get too hot, we may seek water—a cool shower or cold lake—a good balance for the summer heat. Water is the most *yin*, receptive element, the one relating to the emotions. In the body, blue (the color for the Water element) balances red, that is to say, Fire and Water control each other, by keeping each other in balance. They can also injure or attack one another.

If Water is weak, the Fire can rage out of control and lead to heat or inflammation in the body. If Water becomes too strong, it can drown the Fire, and the individual may lose his or her power to act.

The heart and kidney relationship is of key importance in both Western and Chinese medicine. In practice, this Fire and Water relationship correlates with the male (Fire)—female (Water) one. The Fire element relates to sexual energy, and gives life and creative potential, as the sun enables growth and blossoming in nature. The Water element relates to the bladder and kidneys, and rules the sexual organs and their function. Water receives and nourishes, and is also needed for growth.

During sexual intercourse, the male releases Fire (the semen is made from blood and is associated with the Fire element) from his Water element (his kidneys and sex organs) into the female, who receives Fire into her Water element (her sexual organs and womb). Normally, the Fire stimulates the Water (feelings) to move.

So a woman—if the energy of the emotions is not flowing well, or there is too much sexual activity for her—may experience a congestion of energy, of Fire in the pelvic area, and may suffer from inflammation or infection in her sexual organs. In men, too much sexual activity and not enough replenishing can mean that Water takes control over a weakened Fire which can lead to congestion, backaches, and a lack of energy and creativity. It's no joke—we're playing with Fire—so let's learn to understand and use it clearly!

Love is a full circle, giving and receiving all in one. The male ($\male$) in each of us is governed by the Fire (*yang*, active, thrusting) principle while the female ($\female$) in us is ruled by the Water (*yin*, passive, receptive) nature; we each contain both these principles as they are not really separable. This relationship is more between the masculine and feminine principles rather than men and women as individuals. In the male-female relationship, the male/Fire stimulates the Water/feelings in the female, who brings this forth as love through the heart, giving nourishment and love back to the male.

The impulse in relationships is to seek union, joy, and beyond this, to know oneself. However, seeking this communion of spirit, physical union with another may sometimes bring confusion and disenchantment. Physical bodies cannot occupy the same space, yet our soul essences, or spirits, may merge, and all seem to be one. The beauty, contentment, and relaxation from this momentary experience may lead people to seek it time and again through sexual activity.

Eventually, we will see that love is a feeling that arises from within us and goes beyond counter-dependence or people trading the satisfying of their needs with one another. Unattached love, or giving freely, to others as well as to ourselves, can help us understand the differences between love, a body-mind-spirit harmony, and need, an emotional fulfillment. As B. S. ArgIsle states in her poem, "Conditional Love," "Karma (one of the laws of the universe, relating action/reaction, which causes the return of all things to their point of origin) is when we needed each other. Love is when we need nothing."

Mother-Son Law

Speaking of love, an important relationship within the Five Element system is called the Mother-Son law. The body's elements must work together to maintain its fine tuning. This may be seen clearly in the Mother-Son law, or "Creation" cycle. The five elements form a circle in which the mother gives energy to or creates the son and the son receives this energy from the mother.

The cycle thus described is: Fire creates Earth creates Metal creates Water creates Wood creates Fire. For example, spring's Wood and the organs, liver and gall bladder, give energy to summer's Fire, the heart and small intestine. Fire in turn creates Earth, energizing the spleen and stomach.

If the mother element at any point is weak, or unbalanced, it may cause the son element to weaken in turn. Conversely, if the son element is weak, it will demand more from the mother, and weaken her. If the son is congested or has too much energy, this energy may cause the mother's in turn to back up and become congested.

It's all interconnected—in here and out there! We have to keep our channels open and our energy flowing for it all to work properly.

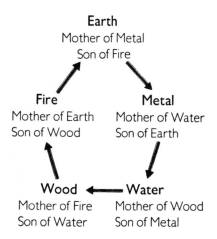

Earth
Mother of Metal
Son of Fire

Fire
Mother of Earth
Son of Wood

Metal
Mother of Water
Son of Earth

Wood
Mother of Fire
Son of Water

Water
Mother of Wood
Son of Metal

Mother-Son Law

Intuition

Intuition is an inner kind of knowing, often called our "sixth sense." It helps us to integrate our inner and outer worlds. It is an important process and can be developed with practice, like anything else.

Intuition has to do with insight (seeing within) and goes along with a receptive state, thus "*yin*-tuition," in which we let the "feelings speak." You do not have to be a meditator or particularly spiritual, but you must allow the thinking mind to become aware of your feelings and other inner senses for this particular knowledge/awareness to emerge into your consciousness.

Intuition is related to the sixth chakra (energy body), the area of the third eye (pineal gland). This ancient light meter, or camera lens of consciousness, is said to open and close depending on how much light you can handle.

Intuition is considered an attribute of the Fire element in the Chinese system as it seems truly to be a sense of the heart; but getting in touch with your intuition actually involves several elements. First, from the Metal, or Air, element, relating to the lungs, you breathe and allow your thinking mind and body to relax. Inspiration means the breathing in of spirit and has to do with being open to the new—ideas, air, nourishment, insights.

Then you will become aware of your feelings (Water) and a flash of light/insight (Fire) will come into your awareness. These sparks of realization can happen anywhere, anytime, if you are open to them. Whether you're sitting quietly by yourself, walking down the street or meeting with friends, this guidance from your heart can be helpful to guide you to your good or protect you from danger.

Our hearts know the truth. If we can learn how to listen for this information, we can answer questions or solve problems that we or others have. We just need to ask and then listen to what our inner knowledge tells us.

We now need to find this fine balance between the heart and the mind. Neither can, or should, take control if you wish to experience good health and continual growth; both have to work together. Keep your mind open and clear, and remember too, as spiritual teacher Parmahansa Yogananda sings, "Listen, listen, listen to your Heart's song."

Summer Diet

Summer is usually hot and we are more active. We need a diet which keeps us cool and light—isn't it fortunate that nature provides us with such luscious fruits and vegetables to eat at this time? The gardens and orchards are full. A diet of primarily raw fruits and vegetables, organically grown (without pesticides and other chemicals), is ideal. This will help you feel lighter, aid in weight loss and keep your energy strong.

Foods have *yin* and *yang* qualities also. Fruits are the most *yin* (wet, cooling) followed by vegetables, whereas the *yang* foods are the more concentrated, heating ones, primarily the proteins (flesh, nuts, seeds, beans), fats (dairy products, eggs), and complex carbohydrates (whole grains). So during the summer eat lots of fresh fruits and juices, multicolored salads and vegetables, some seeds, nuts, and grains, and fewer dairy products and meats.

Obviously, if you are doing physical outdoor work or getting lots of exercise, you need to eat more food. Fruits are good in the morning, early afternoon, or as a nighttime snack, and vegetables then can be eaten more in the latter part of the day. If you eat a heavier meal, you might try to do this in the middle to late afternoon and rest a couple of hours. This will give you overall better evening energy and sleep, plus more complete digestion than eating nearer to bedtime.

One of the Chinese guides to illness suggests that if an organ is unbalanced or overstressed in its season, the difficulty may be expressed in the following season. So summer is not the time to overburden your liver, the main detoxifier for the body. Be careful with fried foods, processed and chemical foods, and drugs of all kinds, especially alcohol, or too much caffeine, as all these can be pollutants with which the liver must deal.

However, if you should overdo it, or have a little too much party drink, the next morning you can start your day with a helpful drink called "Liver Flush," a prescription of Dr. Randolph Stone, father of Polarity Therapy.

To make "Liver Flush" squeeze the juice of one or two lemons (use some seeds and white pulp from the lemon as well), add a tablespoon of cold-pressed olive oil (cold-pressed is hydraulically pressed, not heat-processed), and one or two cloves of garlic (if this is too strong, use a small piece of ginger root). Add a little warm water, blend, and drink first thing in the morning. This is a great tonic and cleanser for the liver.

After drinking this mixture, relax or exercise for a bit, then drink a warm cup of seed tea, either fennel, anise, or fenugreek. Make this by adding two teaspoons of seeds to two cups of water and simmering for 15 minutes in a covered stainless steel, glass, or ceramic pot. Let it sit for another 15 minutes and drink. Aluminum cookware is not recommended as it reacts with foods, possible introducing toxic levels of aluminum into the body. This tea supposedly assists the action of the "Liver Flush" and also acts as a relaxant and carminative (relieves gas) in the digestive system. In another half hour, eat a light breakfast.

Here are a few good breakfast ideas. If you like feeling light, have just a couple pieces of fruit, fruit juice, or tea in the morning. A richer breakfast might include a small bowl of yogurt with one or two sliced pieces of fruit, such as banana, pear, or apple; a few nuts, raisins, and a taste of honey.

You should try not to mix too many different foods together so you can get better digestion and assimilation, and less gas (fermentation of food) in your system. However, everyone's system is a little different, so you need to observe what works best for you.

It seems the body can handle combinations more easily in a blended drink, so here's a high energy, yet light, breakfast that will take you through lunch. For one person (double the amounts for two), add together in a blender two tablespoons of yogurt; one ripe banana, apple, or pear; four ounces of orange or apple juice, or water; one to two tablespoons of

Liver Flush

1–2 lemons
  1 tablespoon cold-pressed
    olive oil
  2 cloves of garlic
  4 ounces spring water

Squeeze the lemons and add the rest of the ingredients to the juice. Blend 30 seconds and drink.

good tasting nutritional (brewer's) yeast (high in B vitamins); one tablespoon of olive oil; and one tablespoon of blackstrap molasses (high in iron and vitamins, and the positive nutritional side of white sugar); blend, and drink up. You can vary the mixture for the flavor and consistency you wish.

A more grounding and heat-producing breakfast, especially on a cold morning or for a day of hard work, could be a bowl of natural dry cereal, like granola, or a cooked one like oats, wheat, or multi-grained cereal with added raisins, sunflower seeds, or nuts, and topped with a little raw milk (nothing taken out or added), or with some almond or coconut milk. With toast, a cup of tea, and maybe a glass of fresh orange juice (for proper food combining to prevent gas, drink 15 minutes before eating), this will give you a good nourished feeling to start the day. Or maybe you only have time for a "Mr. Quickee": a cup of herbal tea with a slice or two of whole grain toast, spread with a nut butter and topped with sliced banana or dates. Be sure to floss and brush your teeth before you go out in a rush.

Foods and the Fire Element

Foods can also be used to replenish the Fire element. Remember, this element relates to the bitter flavor, which is more commonly a taste found in herbs. However, there are a variety of foods considered bitter, which may help nourish your Fire. These include some green leafy vegetables, especially endive, escarole, and watercress; most lettuces have a little of this quality too. Also, coffee, tea, and natural chocolate (without sugar) are bitter, but remember where a little can nourish, too much may cause harm. If the Fire element is too weak or strong, there may be a special attraction or repulsion toward the bitter-flavored foods.

People with increased Fire may be hot types, full of energy, with red complexions, usually very busy; they love to talk and socialize, and may find it hard to relax or to slow down and feel. A cooling diet of primarily fruits and vegetables with lots of juices and water will help. Cucumbers and citrus fruits are especially good.

For people with weak Fire, a more warming and cooked food diet, especially whole grains, may be helpful. Buckwheat and millet are two good heaters. Spices (herbs) like cayenne, ginger, or curry will add a little Fire to the blood.

Diet and the Small Intestine

To receive the nourishment from your food, you must have a properly functioning small intestine. Muramoto, in *Healing Ourselves*, says that a poorly functioning small intestine leads to weak Fire, and thus to poor blood formation. According to herbalist William LeSassier, a good food combination to cleanse and tone the small intestine is equal parts of brown rice, lentils, and sunflower seeds. Add one and a half times the amount of water, and simmer slowly for about 45 minutes. Eat a cup or two daily for a few weeks. It is a tasty, filling dish, and a great heat producer. This should help the assimilation function of the small intestine.

Diet and the Heart

The great advances in medical technology, diagnostics, and surgery, have offered no help to the incidence of heart and vascular disease, nor has a great reduction in the numbers of deaths from these degenerative processes occurred. I believe this is due to the lack of importance placed on preventive education about diet and its effects in the past, and on increased mechanization, reducing daily exercise. The relationship of diet to heart and vascular disease is crucial, and it is finally becoming more widely understood.

Atherosclerosis, the deposit of fats and other debris in the blood vessels, has been associated with high cholesterol and animal fats in the diet. This is also possibly related to a diet high in vegetable (unsaturated) fats found in vegetable oils, seeds, nuts, avocadoes, etc. Deposits, called plaques, in the blood vessels can eventually compromise blood flow and the oxygenation, or life, of the cells and tissues. Acute (short-term) and chronic diseases such as myocardial infarctions (heart attacks), high blood pressure, coronary artery disease, and cerebrovascular accidents (strokes) result from this process.

These diseases may be genetically related, but it is true that types of diets run in families too. My sense is that these problems are in fact more culturally related.

Years of a diet of red meats, animal fats, sugars and starches, along with the additives and preservatives in them, without a regular chance of cleansing the toxins these foods introduce, will clog up the blood vessels. This is especially true for coro-

For an Efficient Small Intestine
Digestion—Assimilation

For Tone
Cook together equal parts of: brown rice, lentils, and sunflower seeds. Eat 1–2 cups daily for 2 weeks. This will also improve body heat.

For Better Function
Rest occasionally from foods.

> "The greatest cause of all heart trouble is a wrong diet, which causes impure blood and weakens the heart . . . other causes are lack of exercise and poor circulation. Often palpitations of the heart are due to gas and fermentation in the stomach.
>
> Many heart problems are caused by tea, coffee, tobacco, and alcoholic liquors. Sometimes heart trouble is caused by too much food made of white flour products, and cane-sugar products. When so much food is eaten that is robbed of its life-giving properties, and since the real health-giving properties that have been refined out of foods are the properties that strengthen our bodies and heart, the heart gets weaker and weaker."
>
> BACK TO EDEN
> *Jethro Kloss*

nary (heart) arteries, where plaques of accumulated fats can lead to inadequate cardiac circulation and thus restricted activity, angina pectoris (pain from insufficient blood flow to the heart), and heart attacks. Low energy, loss of sexual functions, brain/thinking dysfunctions, high blood pressure, kidney problems, and loss of stamina may result from the atherosclerosis throughout the body.

We are learning now that these changes can be reversed through proper diet and exercise. *Live Longer Now* by J. Leonard, J. Hofer, and N. Pritikin, describes the work of the Longevity Research Institute in Santa Barbara, California, and of its director, Nathan Pritikin, who seems to be having some definite success in treating heart disease patients with a program of proper diet and exercise.

A change of diet will change the body state and affect the inherent pathology created from the previous diet. Here are some recommendations from *Live Longer Now* and from my own experience, which are designed to help all stages of heart and vascular diseases. These suggestions may also prevent degenerative diseases from forming. First the "avoidances" and then the "positive actions":

1. *Avoid salt.* Salt is a key villain in the volume-overload aspect of high blood pressure and heated, refined salt with its additives for flow and color is a poison to your body.
2. *Avoid fatty foods* including fried foods. Heated oils are chemically changed making them very hard for the body to digest. Avoid especially fatty meats, oils (you do need a little uncooked, cold-pressed oil in your diet, preferably olive, sesame, or sunflower oils), shortening, butter and dairy products, nuts and avocadoes.
3. *Avoid high cholesterol* foods, particularly eggs (yolks), fatty meats, shellfish and animal organs like liver. If eating meat, only eat small portions of lean meat, poultry (avoid oily skins), or fish.
4. *Avoid sugar* in any of its forms. Avoid all candy, cookies, pastries, packaged cereals, etc. This includes brown sugar, honey, and syrups.
5. *Avoid refined or processed foods, or chemical additives.*
6. *Avoid coffee or caffeine teas.*

Now here are the things you can *do*.

1. *Eat lots of fresh fruit and vegetables*, raw, steamed, or baked. If frying or sauteing foods, try water, not oil.
2. *Eat whole grains* like natural cereals—rolled oats, brown rice, millet, buckwheat, wheat or rye.
3. If needed, eat small amounts of lean meats, poultry, or fish.
4. You can use some vegetable salt, from naturally dried vegetables. Some blends have small amounts of sea salt. Your body needs some salt, and the more you exercise and sweat the more you need. However, if you have heart or blood pressure problems, it is best to avoid even sea salt, soy sauce, and tamari, and obtain the salt you need solely from the foods you eat.
5. *Drink herbal teas.*
6. *Exercise* is a key part.
7. If you start to crave old habits, you might *go for a long walk*, or *take a cold shower!*

A good, wholesome diet, low in fats with adequate exercise and weight control will prevent and alleviate much heart disease.

Depending on your state of health, your body can use some natural, oil-rich foods that you might avoid otherwise in order to keep your fat and oil intake low. These are the seeds like sunflower and sesame, nuts, avocadoes, salad oils, some dairy products, or occasional eggs. Too much of these, however, will be more dietary fat than you need.

Water

In general, most city waters are high in chloride, flouride, and industrial chemicals plus who knows what else, and I recommend using spring water, or purified or distilled water if necessary, for drinking purposes. However, if you must use city tap waters, it's a good idea to boil the water for 15 minutes or to solarize it by placing a clear glass jug filled with water in the sunlight for one to two days before drinking. This takes out much of the chlorine and puts vital energy in—it tastes better too.

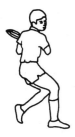

Exercise

Another major factor in keeping the heart and circulatory system, and the whole body in tune, is *exercise.* It also helps strengthen the Fire element. Volumes have been written on all the sports, calisthenics, and practices that help keep the body young and supple. Obviously, you can't do any movement without using your muscles and bones, but you must consider exercise as a separate event from daily work and your household chores and errands. When you take the time and space in your life for a specific activity which takes you to your physical limit and beyond, you will be doing yourself the greatest good.

Exercise to make you sweat will help eliminate some toxins from the blood through the skin. Sweat is a by-product of the circulatory process in which capillaries bring heat (blood flow) to the skin and dump waste products. Daily exercise up to your *own* limits will open up the old circulation and create new "collateral" circulation. "Collaterals" refer to new blood vessels which form and grow to provide more blood flow to needed areas which have had restricted circulation. This is vital to people with heart and blood vessel disease who need increased circulation. Regular exercise is a stimulus for the formation of collateral blood vessels.

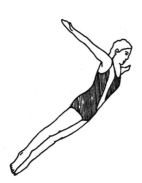

Exercise will alleviate tiredness and lack of energy as well as reduce excessive weight by increasing energy output. It aids elimination both by sweating and by stimulating the functions of the internal organs and the intestines. Exercise can also help increase strength, endurance, and coordination. It aids in reducing stress, and providing a sense of well-being, as well as improving flexibility and reducing joint and muscular stiffness.

As if the previous advantages aren't enough, my belief is that exercise slows down the aging process and promotes longevity—but it takes work and commitment to keep yourself in top shape. It also may be addictive as you feel better when you do it than when you miss it.

Obviously, different exercise programs can be geared toward different goals. Weight-lifting, isometrics (working muscle groups against themselves), and calisthenics will help increase muscle size, tone, and strength. Jogging and running, swimming, and other sports aid strength and also improve lung capacity and endurance. They can give you more stamina

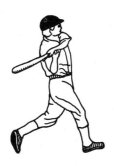

to deal with life. Stretching exercises, such as yoga and the martial art forms like aikido, kung fu, or tai chi, will aid in flexibility and coordination, promote strength and mental/ physical relaxation, and are a good internal balance for the more active, outward sports.

The *Royal Canadian Air Force: Exercise Plans for Physical Fitness* promotes its program by the motto, "Feel better—look better—now." It states simply that "physical fitness is a direct result of the physical activity; physical activity leading to physical fitness must be vigorous and regular; and people *will* accept challenge." Its exercise program is primarily stretching and calisthenics and regular practice will "increase muscle tone, muscular strength, muscular endurance, flexibility, and the efficiency of your heart." However, it goes on to state that fitness is a personal thing, each of us being our own best judge of what fitness is and what it means to us.

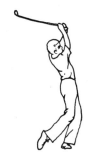

Exercise is used in weight control, in relieving chronic tiredness, and in helping minor aches and pains. Here are some "pertinent facts" paraphrased from the *Royal Canadian Air Force* book:

1. Muscles not adequately exercised or used become weak and inefficient.
2. Weak back muscles are a major source of low back pains and increasing their strength will help eliminate these pains.
3. The efficiency and capacity of our lungs, heart, and other organs can be improved by *regular vigorous* exercise.
4. A fit person is less susceptible to common injuries, and if injured, recovers more rapidly.
5. The incidence of degenerative heart diseases may be greater in those who have not followed a physically active life.
6. Regular vigorous exercise plays an important role in controlling our weight and in helping us to reduce emotional and nervous tension.
7. We are never too old to begin and follow a regular exercise program.

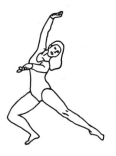

My main interest is to get you inspired and out there "doing it," appreciating the importance of regular exercise. If you think you are too busy, or have other excuses, you need to re-evaluate your life priorities. If you think you are too old, too tired, too sick—you just have to get started at your own capacity.

My health coach says "Do it—if you're hungry, exercise; if you're tired, exercise, eat and rest later!!!" Exercise will use up that fat that would be stored during inactivity; and excessive fats and sugars circulating in the blood can cause tiredness.

With all these benefits, there are more. Regular exercise actually plays a part in preventing and reversing the degenerative diseases. In *Live Longer Now*, many studies are quoted to show the positive effects of exercise on heart disease, high blood pressure, and diabetes, but it can also help prevent many illnesses. It will help you feel younger and add vitality to your days and years to your life, and especially influence those middle years, ages 40–60. Remember, "You are as young as you feel."

Aerobics also offers many healthful exercise programs. In his book, *The New Aerobics*, Kenneth Cooper, M.D. writes, "Aerobics refers to a variety of exercises that stimulate heart and lung activity for a time period sufficiently long to produce beneficial changes in the body. Running, swimming, cycling, jogging—these are typical aerobic exercises. There are many others."

Aerobics gets you to work at your own capacity, which, as you become a regular participant in your program, will increase. Be aware of factors such as your age, physical condition and any illness, especially heart and lung problems. It is a good idea to have a complete medical evaluation before you begin any strenuous exercise program, particularly if you have some illness or are over 30 years old.

Aerobics are important to maintain heart health and to remedy problems. You can create a daily, weekly, or monthly program to provide you with the regularity and variety you wish. Some people like to pick one activity and do it every day, while others may get bored and need diversity. A good time to exercise is before or after a work day, to help reduce or relieve stress and provide a sense of well-being. It is much better for you than a couple of drinks to relax after a hard day at the office.

There is such a wide range of possibilities that I will only offer a few guidelines. One hour a day is important to devote to your own fitness. At least 30 minutes is devoted to vigorous exercise that promotes sweating, 15 minutes to mild exercise and 15 minutes to stretching. It is important to loosen and stretch your muscles before vigorous activities to help prevent injuries. Realize that this is a program for a healthy, active person. If you are very overweight, ill, or just beginning to exercise, start more slowly, yet one hour per day is a good goal. Go at your own speed.

A crash exercise program, like crash diets, is not particularly helpful and may be dangerous. Have a good time. Exercise should be fun. It's a chance to be with yourself—your body, your feelings, your mind, breath, and environment. Make a deal with yourself and start your program. You can only win!

Herbs

Summer is the season to strengthen your Fire element if it is weak. Lots of sun will help, as will exercise, good foods and good elimination. There are also a couple common herbs that can be used safely for this.

Cayenne pepper (*Capsicum annum*) is one of nature's true stimulants, and medicinally, is known as a tonic, alterative, pungent, stimulant and sialogogue. It provides quick energy and though it acts as a heating agent, it is not irritating. It has been applied to wounds and sores and used for an irritated or ulcerated stomach or colon. Cayenne has also been applied as a liniment or poultice for rheumatism, joint inflammations, and gum problems.

Cayenne pepper is actually the fruit or pod of the plant. It is very high in vitamin C. This, with its stimulating and heating effects, makes it a good herb for colds, flus and sore throats, plus weak circulation and cold or damp feet. Cayenne pepper is a heart stimulant as well, and acts as a blood cleanser, that is, it helps to eliminate impurities from the blood by increasing urine flow or sweating. It has also been used to treat problems of the kidneys, spleen, and pancreas.

As a stimulant, cayenne can either be taken as capsules, two to three, several times daily, or as a half teaspoon mixed into a glass of water. For its tonic effects, two capsules taken twice daily for 30–60 days will help strengthen your circulation and cleanse your blood. The bright red "African bird pepper" is the best to use rather than the light orange varieties.

Ginger root (*Zingiber officinale*) is another common herb. It

Solar or Lunar Tea

Place dry or fresh herbs in a clear glass jug and put it in the Sun/ Moon for one to two days/ nights—then drink or refrigerate.

Aromatic leaf herbs or flowers work best.

Examples:
Peppermint leaf
Hibiscus flowers
Lemon grass
Red clover flowers
Chamomile flowers
Any green herbs
Rosemary
Orange or lemon peel

acts as a stimulant, pungent, carminative, aromatic, sialogogue, and when taken hot, as a diaphoretic. It works more slowly than cayenne pepper but is very good for circulation, and both these herbs help increase body Fire. Ginger root has also been used for suppressed menstruation, colds, sore throats, diarrhea, indigestion and nausea. Add 6–8 thin slices of ginger root to two cups of boiling water and simmer 15–20 minutes. Drink a cup or two daily for a month and observe the effects that this has on your body heat and circulation.

Hot greens like mustard, watercress, cauliflower, or cabbage will also stimulate the Fire; while garlic in your diet is good for strong, clean blood, and will ward off any vampires (friends too for that matter). Herbalist William LeSassier offers a formula for strengthening the blood, which in turn helps the heart. Combine equal parts of nettle, dulse, chives, watercress, and yellow dock root, either in a soup or dried and powdered to sprinkle as a seasoning taste tonic. This and other blood cleansers are good also for chronic skin problems, and some acute ones, like staphylococcal sores (impetigo, boils), which seem related to impure blood. Impure blood is a naturopathic concept, seeing blood as impure when it has substances in it, such as chemicals, microorganisms, or other impurities, which are not usually present. These must be eliminated from the blood via its primary routes, or secondarily through the skin. Red clover blossoms, steeped as a tea, is another of the herbal blood cleansers and a good summertime herb.

If you become too hot (too much Fire), you could get into the shade, jump in the water, have some cooling fruit juices like orange juice or lemonade, and try some cooling herbs. These are mostly the green herbs like mints and many of the flowers, such as hibiscus and chamomile flowers. Boil some water and pour it into a pot with one or several of these herbs and let them steep for 20–30 minutes.

Never boil greens or flowers as their aromatic oils and other essentials will be lost. For hot weather, make some iced tea by adding ice or refrigerating your brew before drinking. With a little honey or maple syrup, it's a great summer treat.

All of these herbs can be made as "solar teas" by placing some herb in a glass jug with water and leaving it out in the sunlight for a day. For you moon babies, make some lunar teas near full moon by leaving the jug with herbs and water out in the moonlight for one or two nights.

Small Intestine Herbs

Some specific herbs for the small intestine include comfrey root, licorice root, fennel seed and anise seed. Comfrey root acts as a tonic and healer to the intestinal lining when used daily for one to two months. Boil one tablespoon of root in two cups of water for 20 minutes and drink one to two cups daily.

For intestinal gas or indigestion, fennel or anise tea is helpful. Simmer one teaspoon per cup for 15 minutes and drink several times daily. Licorice root, the "great peacemaker," helps soothe the digestive system and is a mild laxative; it is also a nice herb for children. It is a soft root, so simmering one teaspoon per cup for 10 minutes should extract its essence.

Helpful Herbs

Simmer one tablespoon comfrey root in two cups of water for 20 minutes. Drink 1–2 cups daily for 30 days. This will tonify, clear, and strengthen the intestinal mucous lining.

Fennel or anise seed—simmer one teaspoon per cup for 10 minutes, then steep for 15 minutes. Used for gas or indigestion.

Herbs and the Heart

Herb care for the heart is a more difficult subject. Some herbs are strong and must be used carefully, and many others are not very effective. Most herbalists don't treat the heart directly (this is also true for acupuncturists) but strengthen and clean the blood or do a general tonification of the organ systems.

Digitalis, the key heart drug used today, is made from the foxglove plant, which has strong cardiac-stimulating properties and should be used only in skilled hands. Lily of the valley is another cardiac stimulant, and like digitalis, should be used with care. However, there are some herbs which are safe and effective.

Hawthorn berries have been used by herbalists as a heart tonic both in structural and physiological heart disorders. Dr. Edward Shook says, "It is a diuretic, astringent, and tonic, also used for sore throat, and as a diuretic in dropsy (congestive heart failure) and kidney troubles." Boil one quart of water and pour this over two ounces of hawthorn berries and let steep in the pot for 30 minutes. Drink a cup twice daily or one half cup four times daily.

Another herb that is a general tonic and rejuvenator and is known to strengthen the heart is ginseng root. This ancient oriental herb is a growing panacea for those seeking youthful strength as it stimulates the nervous and endocrine systems, enhancing stamina and virility. American ginseng root is growing in quality and popularity. The root takes a minimum

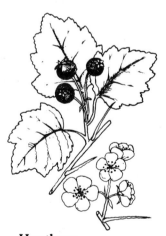

Hawthorn
Crateegos oxyacawtha

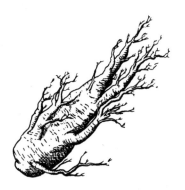

Ginseng
Panax quinquefolia

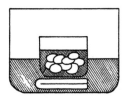

Preparing Ginseng Tea

of six years to mature; some Chinese or Korean roots that are 50–100 years old are available.

I recommend preparing ginseng root "Chinese" style. This involves double boiling for 6 to 8 hours. Place the sliced root in a small glass jar or ceramic pot then pour in two cups of boiling water and cover. Place this into a larger pot with water and let the water simmer for 6–8 hours, watching water levels. If you place the jar on the bottom of the pot, put it on top of a small cloth or towel to keep the ginseng water from boiling or the jar from breaking in case the water goes too low. Drink one cup before bed and the second cup upon arising the next morning.

Ginseng is a very *yang* root, so it is a builder and it is suggested that no fruit or vegetables (*yin* foods) be eaten for 2–3 days while using the ginseng root. Many Oriental people use ginseng daily as a rejuvenator. Extracts and powders are available that can be used to make a daily tea. However, a really good root could be used monthly, at the beginning of each season, or once a year. This herb is used primarily for men, though women use it, too. However, it may be too strong to recommend during pregnancy.

The borage plant (*Borago officinalis*), leaves or flowers, is another herb that can strengthen the heart, but it seems to work more on the emotional level, bringing happiness. The flowers especially can be eaten or made as tea, and have been used for centuries to help with melancholy and just forgetting your troubles.

Other cardiac herbs are motherwort, asparagus, golden seal, peppermint, tansy, sorrel, and valerian root.

Color Therapy

Those interested in using specific color vibrations for balancing the body systems, can prepare solarized, color-energized waters by leaving water in the sunlight in colored glass bottles for a couple of days. From this you will receive predominantly that color vibration in your water. Drinking this water can actually be used to balance certain disharmonies, though subtle it may be. For summer, the cooling blue and green bottles are good to keep available.

Color therapy has been used since the beginning of time. Indeed, we use it daily in the clothes we choose to wear, in the foods we eat, and in the colors with which we surround ourselves. But there is also a specific form of treatment which associates each ailment as a certain color imbalance. By the use of a white light shown through colored gels, the parts of the body affected are color-treated.

Stanley Burroughs' *Healing for the Age of Enlightenment* is one of the books on the market that discusses color therapy.

The following chart describes some of the associations, actions, and problems that have been treated by the seven colors of the rainbow.

The seven chakras are also known as the seven energy bodies, the storehouses of the different powers of the whole being. As in the acupuncture system, all mental, emotional, and physical symptoms can be seen as manifestations of specific congestions or weaknesses within the corresponding chakras.

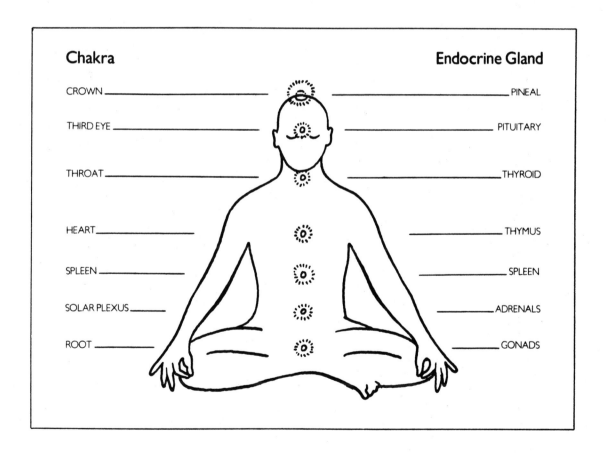

Chakra	Endocrine Gland
CROWN	PINEAL
THIRD EYE	PITUITARY
THROAT	THYROID
HEART	THYMUS
SPLEEN	SPLEEN
SOLAR PLEXUS	ADRENALS
ROOT	GONADS

Color	Musical Note	Chakra (Energy Body) Location/Function/ Behavior	Color's Effect	Problems Treated
Red	C	1st—base of spine creative, sexual and restorative process transmutation	energizes, vitalizes, heats, and promotes circulation; stimulates adrenalin, red blood cell production, menstrual flow and sexual power; strengthens willpower and courage	anemia infertility/impotence colds and chills weak menstruation (not in fevers or nervous problems)
Orange	D	2nd—below navel emotional center purification	warms and cheers, frees bodily and emotional tension; aids mentality	lung ailments epilepsy mental problems rheumatism kidney troubles
Yellow	E	3rd—solar plexus thinking (mental) center ambition	inspires and awakens the mind; strengthens the nerves; helps reasoning, aids self control; aids elimination; improves skin; a cerebral and nerve stimulant	stomach troubles indigestion, gas, constipation liver problems eczema nervous exhaustion
Green	F	4th—heart area sensitivity—feelings compassion/harmony	harmonizes and balances, soothes and restores; a tonic; stimulates the heart; soothes the nerves, brain, heart, and eyes; helps elimination; refreshes	headaches heart ailments ulcers eye problems nervous conditions
Blue	G	5th—throat area communication self-expression	antiseptic, cooling, sedative, relaxing, and soothing; helps stop bleeding; helps with nutrition and building the skin and body; promotes truth, loyalty, and reliability	all inflammations throat problems fevers, infections burns spasms, pain headaches, diarrhea
Indigo	A	6th—pineal (pituitary area) (third eye) perception realization	electric, cooling, astringent; anaesthetic effect; builds white blood cells; increases activity of the spleen; depresses heart and nervous system	pneumonia mental problems convulsions eye, ear, and nose problems
Violet	B	7th—crown (top of head) universal consciousness oneness	stimulates spiritual nature and intuition; elevates inspiration; expands divine understanding	mental disorders neuroses neuralgia concussions cramps tumors scalp problems

For Heart Health, here's the *Heart Head:*

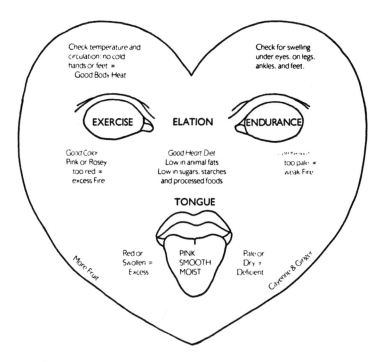

Summary

Following the rains of winter and spring which prepare the earth, the brilliant sunshine of summer allows nature to flourish. We tend to and watch the garden grow and mature from the seeds we planted months before. The garden image may apply to whatever projects we begin; if we continue to put energy into them like sun, water, care, love—they grow and we all prosper. This relates to plants, children, relationships, and work. If we do not continue to nourish them, they may wilt and perish.

The summer is associated with the Fire element in the Chinese system. The organs ruled by this element are the heart and small intestine as well as the functions of circulation and heating in the body.

Diet and exercise are very important to keeping the Fire element strong. Proper nutrition is vital to maintaining a healthy heart and for providing fuel and heat for the body. So our diet could be changed by eliminating refined foods, tea, coffee, alcohol, and tobacco, and by cutting down on animal fats, particularly red meats, dairy products, and other fatty foods. Most heart troubles can be overcome, especially if you don't wait too long. It is also true that it takes time, commitment, and hard work to undo illnesses that have taken years to develop.

The small intestine absorbs the nutrients from foods we eat to feed every cell through good blood circulation. And exercise provides that good blood circulation.

Exercise is also important. An hour a day is little to ask for the benefit you will get from exercise, and the summer is a good time to start. If you are already doing it, you can increase your efforts, your goals, and your well-being in this summer sunshine.

"The body is a machine, you gotta keep it clean and oiled or 'twill spoil."

B.S. ArgIsle

You have a new car to start driving around—it's your body. Get it out of the garage, shine it up, and take it for a spin. You may even realize you have a third and fourth gear. If it appears to need a little tune-up, get it checked; but often just driving it will have it purring in no time. Remember to feed it lots of light, wholesome fuel this summer. Fresh fruits and vegetables, lots of water and juice, big salads, and some whole grains will all give it the power it needs.

Summer is a time to recharge those internal batteries with solar power. Keep the Fire balanced with Water inside and out, and keep the body loose, getting good exercise. It is a time for growth and coming forth. It's a season for good times too, and vacations. For many, it's a season to prepare for going back to school or work.

夏

Summer

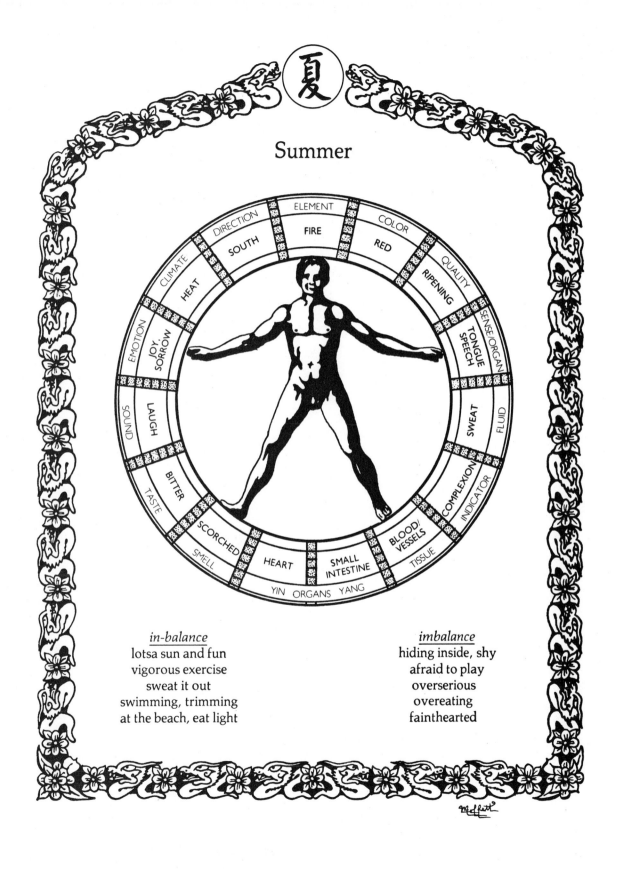

ELEMENT
FIRE

DIRECTION
SOUTH

COLOR
RED

CLIMATE
HEAT

QUALITY
RIPENING

EMOTION
JOY, SORROW

SENSE/ORGAN
TONGUE SPEECH

SOUND
LAUGH

SWEAT

FLUID

TASTE
BITTER

COMPLEXION
INDICATOR

SMELL
SCORCHED

HEART

SMALL INTESTINE

BLOOD/ VESSELS

TISSUE

YIN ORGANS YANG

in-balance
lotsa sun and fun
vigorous exercise
sweat it out
swimming, trimming
at the beach, eat light

imbalance
hiding inside, shy
afraid to play
overserious
overeating
fainthearted

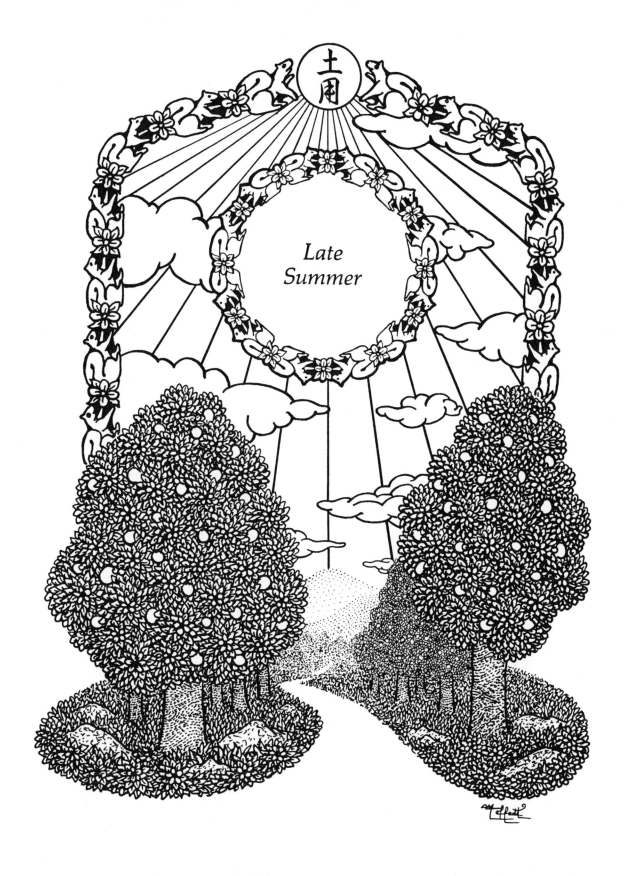

Late Summer: Seasonal Transitions

IN THE FIVE ELEMENT THEORY, there are five seasons whose nature is related to the five elements. Late summer is correlated with the element Earth. It is an important element, and even though it is a short season, it gets its own section in this book.

Late summer, or "Indian summer," is that special time at the end of summer and before autumn, when there is often a glorious "hot spell." This is also an important period of preparation and readiness for the year's work. Nature is rich and full, apples and corn and harvests galore; for us, it is back to school or work, and making new plans.

The fertile and stable Earth we know as our Mother not only gives us the food that we eat—the Earth is our support on which we stand and lay ourselves to rest: our womb and our tomb. Being earthy or grounded is having our roots in a solid base. The Earth, revolving around its axis to make a day, relates to the cycles in nature, in man and woman, and is central to all the other elements.

In the Chinese system, the center is the direction associated with the Earth element; we are all around it and it surrounds us. It is also called "doyo" in Chinese, meaning "transition," so this element relates to the times of seasonal change which come four times a year (rather than just the summer-autumn transition) for about two-three weeks each, around the two solstices and the two equinoxes.

Late summer itself is a short season, but it can be a time of

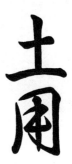

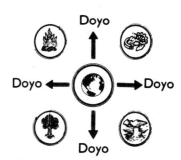

intense metamorphosis in nature and within ourselves. This period of time has some aspects of all the seasons and often weather which is very hot, cold, or some other extreme, occurs at these times of "doyo." During transitional periods, it is especially important to stay centered, a state of being in contact with the Earth that we call "grounded," so as not to go into total chaos. If things are in motion, both inwardly and outwardly, there is nothing to hold onto.

Earth Element

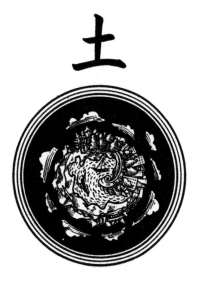

A quotation from ancient Chinese texts taken from *Healing Ourselves* describes some associations for the Earth Element.

"The Center creates Humidity; humidity nourishes the Earth; the forces of the Earth create humidity in Heaven and Fertile Soil upon Earth. They create the Stomach organ and the Flesh within the body . . . And the Mouth, and the Yellow color and the Sweet flavor . . . The emotion Sympathy, and the ability to Sing."

A strong attraction or dislike for one of these, such as the yellow color or a humid climate, may in turn be a clue to an imbalance in the Earth element. If a yellowish hue is seen in the face and around the eyes, this could mean that there is a problem in the Earth element. This is different from jaundice.

When the emotion of sympathy or compassion, for example, is dominant, this may also reflect an Earth problem. We may then find that we need a great deal of sympathy from others and might even create illness or difficulties to get the attention we require. The other side of this imbalance is not being able to receive sympathy or give it at all.

The Earth element gives us the power of manifestation. From the action of Fire comes the product of Earth. The materialization of money through labor of mind or body, the writing of words to create a book, or the drawing or photography of an artist to produce visual images, are all examples of this process. What these products say to others, or how we use them are aspects of communication, which is represented by the next element, Metal.

The Earth element also gives us the ability to form thoughts, views, and opinions. An imbalance of this element may show itself mentally as a tendency toward obsession, going over and over certain ideas or problems, which can even be obstinancy or stubborness toward accepting new ideas, viewpoints, or life changes. This type of thinking may have an adverse effect on the digestive organs, and can lead to indigestion and belching, also associated with an Earth element imbalance.

This element gives one the ability to make the singing sound, and someone whose speaking voice is strong in this quality may have an imbalance of the Earth energy. The associated smell for the Earth element is fragrant.

Since this element relates to the intake of nourishment, it seems appropriate that the sense organ is the mouth, the sense associated with the Earth is taste, and the body fluid is saliva. In fact, one may look at the lips (the "indicator" of this element) as an indication of the health of the Earth element. If problems like swelling, cracking, or peeling are present, they may suggest an imbalance in this element.

The throat is also under the influence of the Earth element, as is the flesh, which means everything between our skin and our muscles, medically called the subcutaneous, or "soft" tissue. Many Chinese texts say that the Earth rules the muscles as well, so problems there such as pain or stiffness may suggest an improper function of this element. Other correspondences for the Earth element are the grain millet, the fruit date, and the green herb mallow, while the animal meat is beef or ox. It is possible that these foods may be particularly nourishing for the Earth element and that too much of these could cause an imbalance.

The spleen and stomach are the body organs connected with the Earth element. In Chinese medicine, the spleen is a central organ, both physiologically and anatomically, and defects in its energy can affect the whole body. The spleen distributes the energy obtained from foods through the body. The other organs depend on it for life. According to the *Nei Ching*, "The five viscera all desire their breath of life from the Spleen; it is the Spleen that is the foundation of existence of the five viscera." The spleen governs the will, the memory, and the ability to form opinions. If the spleen is malfunctioning, there may be a loss of "strength of will" and one may "seem foolish." Spleen trouble may cause forgetfulness and worry.

The Earth element relates to the cycles in nature and within us. In women, it governs the menstrual cycle—the regularity, ease of flow and amount of blood. If these are fine it may

"Stomach is the official of the public granaries and grants the five tastes. . . . (it) acts as a place of accumulation for water and grain and as a source of supply for the six bowels."
NEI CHING

"The spleen and stomach are sentries guarding the governmental storage rooms."
CHINESE FOLK MEDICINE

"The spleen is the ruler over the end of summer, which is conceived of as a season by itself. It's condition may be read from a person's lips; if injured, whiteness will appear in the region of the mouth. It acts upon the flesh and muscles and belongs to that essence of yin *which penetrates the aura of the earth."*
CHINESE FOLK MEDICINE

Stomach Meridian

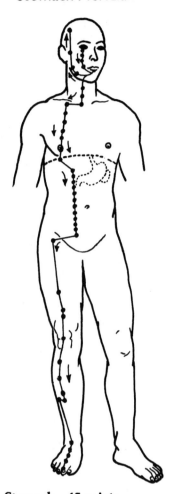

Stomach—45 points
The stomach meridian begins on the face under the eye and runs by the mouth onto the jaw and temple, then down the neck onto the chest, then parallel to the center line of the body, down the outside of the thigh and calf, then along the center top of the foot, and ends at the outside of the second toenail.

Note: Meridians run on both sides of the body

suggest that the spleen is near balance, and conversely, if there are problems in this cycle, such as irregularity, pain, or scanty or excessive bleeding, the spleen or Earth element may be too weak or strong. The Earth gives us fertileness. Problems of infertility are associated often with an Earth element imbalance.

Traditional Chinese philosophy teaches that the stomach is the receiver of nourishment, taking the energy from food for the spleen to distribute. The sensitive stomach has to do with "stomaching" things, that is, being able to tolerate or digest; this relates to food but also to other aspects of life, like thoughts or feelings. If the stomach is working improperly, we may be poorly nourished and weak. The way in which we nourish ourselves and are able to give and receive love and compassion are very important to the health of the Earth element—the stomach and spleen.

The spleen, stomach, and Earth element rule the Center, which nourishes the four corners of the Earth, the four directions. The Earth element plays an important role during transition times, and seasonal changes. During these times, it is most important to stay centered.

Stomach and Digestion

The stomach, spleen and pancreas (the pancreas is associated with the spleen in the Chinese system) are the organs which take their energy from the Earth element. They are essential for the digestive process.

The digestive organs and their functioning reflect the influences of diet, mental activity, and emotions. In fact, the stomach may be one of the most sensitive organs in the body. The whole digestive system is finely tuned by the nervous system, so stress of any kind affects its function. For example, the nerves govern the secretions of acids and enzymes, and the movements of the digestive organs. By speeding up or slowing down the transit foods, the nervous system controls the assimilation of nutrients. Jittery nerves, apprehension, or over-excitement can cause the rapid passage of food and thus, diarrhea, when you do not have time to assimilate your nutrients. The slowing down of intestinal motility from uptightness, resistance, anger, or "holding on" can lead to constipation, where you over-absorb water and toxins from the colon back into the body.

The way the body is processing your food shows up in your moment-to-moment energy state. Taking care with your diet, chewing well, eating a reasonable amount of food in a relaxed setting will all do you good. Bombarding your body with chemical pollutants, or eating too many foods at one time, or eating too fast, or gulping your food down on the run—you pay for it!

The state of your emotions is closely linked to your eating habits and your ability to process food. Being emotionally upset or under stress at all affects your appetite and your nourishment, while feeling happy and clear stimulates your hunger, digestive ability, utilization and appreciation of foods. In our Western culture, the ability to relax, sit, and savor a meal without overeating is often a sign of a contented, healthy human being.

The stomach receives the nourishment and prepares it for further digestion, while the spleen and pancreas, according to the Oriental model, oversee the distribution of nourishment throughout the body. Just as the whole body needs a balance of both activity and rest, so does the digestive tract. Over-activity from too much, or too frequent, eating will overwork, weaken, and even wear out the digestive system. You may even find that it breaks down to get the rest it needs.

After eating and then a short spell of relaxation, the body needs to move a bit, take a walk or dance lightly. This movement aids the digestion, assimilation, and distribution of nutrients.

The mouth is the sense organ associated with the Earth element, and the functions of chewing and the initial enzymatic breakdown of foods are vital to good digestion. The stomach in turn is the abdominal recipient of the chewed and swallowed intake. In response, it adds hydrochloric acid and other digestive juices, consisting of enzymes like pepsin and rennin which help break down protein and milk products. The stomach also helps mix and churn the foods by its muscle-wall activity.

More enzymes and other substances to break down the foods are also secreted by the salivary glands, by the pancreas, the gall bladder (bile), and the small intestine (see chart) to help change the foods into the simple, usable components which then travel through the intestines where they are absorbed by the blood.

Spleen Meridian

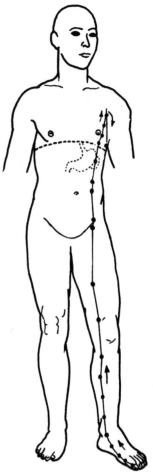

Spleen—21 points
The spleen meridian begins by the nail of the big toe, runs along the instep of the foot and onto the calf and thigh, then the groin, up the abdomen, along the chest lateral to the nipple, up to the axilla, then ends at the side of the chest in the 5th intercostal space.

Note: Meridians run on both sides of the body

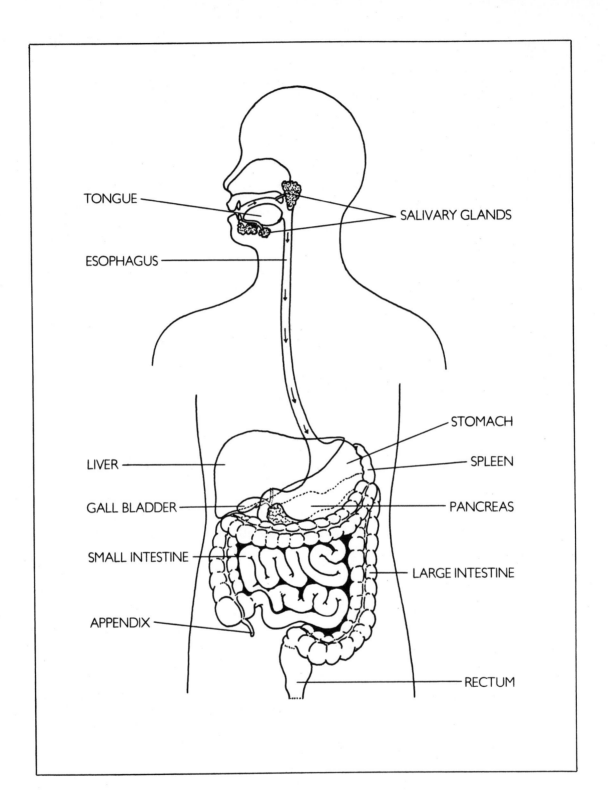

TONGUE

SALIVARY GLANDS

ESOPHAGUS

STOMACH

LIVER

SPLEEN

GALL BLADDER

PANCREAS

SMALL INTESTINE

LARGE INTESTINE

APPENDIX

RECTUM

Digestion Chart

Organ	Substance	Acts on	End Product
Mouth (Salivary Glands)	salivary amylase* (ptaylin)	starch	maltose
Stomach	pepsin	protein	polypeptides
	rennin	casein of milk	milk coagulates
	hydrochloric acid	creates digestive media	
Duodenum (First part of Small Intestine)	secretin	stimulates flow of pancreatic juice	
	pancreozymin	stimulates production of enzymes	
Pancreas	amylase	starch, glycogen	maltose
	lipase	emulsified fats	fatty acids and glycerol
	proteases (trypsin, chymotrypsin, carboxypeptidase)	proteins	protein fragments and amino acids
	ribonuclease and deoxyribonuclease	nucleic acids	polynucleotides
Small Intestine	enterokinase	activates trypsinogen	trypsin
	maltase	maltose	glucose
	sucrase	sucrose	glucose, fructose
	lactase	lactose	glucose, galactose
	proteases	protein fragments	amino acids
	lecithinase	lecithin	glycerol, fatty acids, phosphoric acid, and choline
Liver/Gall Bladder	bile salts	large fat globules	emulsified fats, fatty acids, and bile salt coagulates

*Enzymes end in the letters "ase" and are proteins that act to help catalyze a chemical reaction which changes one substance into another.

Food-Combining

Food-combining involves the proper mixing or separation of foods at meals for the best digestion and for extracting as much nutrition as possible. Given the basic American eating habits, proper food-combining may appear to be a fanatic indulgence contrary to the popular concept of a "balanced meal." We don't stop to think that a meal which provides too many foods is actually an unbalanced meal and can lead to faulty digestion, poor absorption, and fermentation in the bowels. It is no surprise that the great industry of dietary aids for the "tummy" and the "seltzers" for gas and indigestion accompany our usual eating habits. The concept of balancing your diet over the whole day allows simpler food preparation, easier digestion, and better nutritional assimilation.

As you can see on the "Digestion Chart," there are different digestive substances, which break down each kind of food, suggesting, according to food physiologists, that each food has its own best media, as well as stimulating the release of the acids and enzymes it needs for its own complete digestion. Certain foods need very little hydrochloric acid while others need a lot, and some foods you eat can interfere with the breakdown of other foods. For instance, acidic fruits disturb the effectiveness of certain enzymes, such as the amylases, needed to digest starches, so that eating fruits together with starches may inhibit starch digestion.

We should consider the possibility that nature provided us with a system which appreciates simplicity and not mixing our foods. Another possibility is that foods which grow together may be eaten together.

All foods eaten at the same time must be broken down to the same consistency before the stomach will actually begin emptying. But fats and proteins take longer to digest than do carbohydrates. For example, simple fruits may take 10 to 20 minutes, while meats can take 45 to 90 minutes, depending on how well they are chewed. If fruits are eaten at the same time as meat, they will then have an extra hour in the stomach. During this time, fermentation will take place, introducing gas into the system and causing indigestion, belching, and/or cramps.

There is a "flow-chart" on page 103 which demonstrates good food-combining for the best digestion. Foods within the same categories are best eaten together, although what mixes well for us as individuals may vary. A simple list of foods in order of decreasing ease of digestibility and increasing length of time in the stomach includes: fruits, vegetables, grains, beans, seeds, nuts, dairy products, and meats.

Proper food-combining over a whole day might start with fruit in the early morning. If you wish to have a grain cereal or other protein for breakfast, you might eat this a half-hour after the fruit. For lunch you could have salad, vegetables, a milk

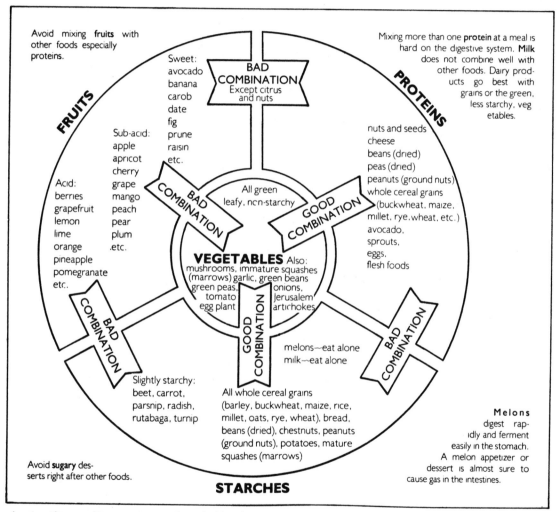

A scientific set of instructions as founded by the Natural Hygiene Institute and Herbert Shelton for non-fermenting properly digesting food combinations.

product, meat, or a grain; they all combine together fairly well. For dinner, a whole grain with cooked vegetables and/or a raw salad gives you a lot of food, filling and nourishing, which will digest well. Meat, cheese, or egg dishes instead of a grain or bean will also combine well with vegetables or a salad.

Fruits in the morning and vegetables in the afternoon is a motto I follow, but a fruit snack in the evening or before bed works better than eating any heavier foods. Vegetables combine well with most other foods and are alkaline-forming.

Acid and Alkaline Diets

There is a lot of talk about "mucus-less diets" and about acid or alkaline diets. Each food when metabolized in the body breaks down into acid or alkaline elements. The body is normally slightly alkaline, the blood pH being 7.41.

Mucus is considered to be related to acid-forming foods, also called mucus-forming foods. We need some mucus for body function. However, if a diet too high in acid-forming foods is eaten, the body can become too acidic and will produce excessive mucus which can be the medium conducive for the growth of bacteria and viruses. Excess mucus can create congestion, the cause of so many illnesses. The body's attempt to remedy this problem of congestion by the elimination of the excessive mucus and acid elements such as through colds, sinus problems or skin rashes is often mistakingly seen as the illness. The problem lies more in the diet.

Interestingly, the acid-alkaline action is not necessarily related to how foods taste. For example, citrus fruits taste acidic, but they are alkaline forming and are good to eat. Other alkaline foods include the grains buckwheat and millet, lima and soy beans; honey; and seed and vegetable oils. Most protein foods—meats and other animal and sea beings; eggs and milk products; butter and cream; nuts and nut oils; seeds and many of the grains; and sugars—are all acid-forming in the body. A diet which consists of 70 to 80 percent alkaline-forming foods will keep the eliminative and nervous systems strong, and you will feel able to work and relax easily, with your entire body in harmony. This means eating lots of fruits and vegetables.

Colds and infections, and even chronic degenerative diseases, will diminish as you move toward a more alkaline diet. Even if you are not sick, you will notice a beneficial change. Try it and see for yourself.

Acid and Alkaline Foods

The body seems to work best on a diet high in alkaline-forming foods—those foods which give alkaline elements when broken down by the digestion. A diet which contains 70%–80% alkaline-forming foods is ideal for healthful living.

Fruits
Acid
cranberries
pomegranates
strawberries
sour fruits

Alkaline
apples
bananas
citrus fruits
dates
grapes
cherries
peaches
pears
plums
papaya
mangoes
pineapple
raspberries
blackberries
huckleberries
elderberries
boysenberries
persimmons
apricots
olives
coconut
figs
raisins
melons

Vegetables
All vegetables are alkaline (includes starchy vegetables like potatoes, squash and parsnips.)

Grains
Acid
Brown Rice
Barley
Wheat
Oats
Rye
Breads

Alkaline
Millet
Buckwheat
Corn
Sprouted grains

Meats and Dairy Products
Acid
All meats
Fish
Fowl
Eggs
Cheese
Milk
Yogurt
Butter

Alkaline
Non-fat milk

Nuts
Acid
Cashews
Walnuts
Filberts
Peanuts
Pecans
Macadamia nuts

Alkaline
Almonds
Brazil nuts

Seeds
Acid
Pumpkin
Sesame
Sunflower
Chia
Flax

Alkaline
All sprouted seeds

Beans and Peas
Acid
Lentils
Navy
Aduki
Kidney

Alkaline
Soybeans
Limas
Sprouted beans

Sugars
Acid
Brown sugar
White sugar
Milk sugar
Cane syrup
Malt syrup
Maple syrup
Molasses

Alkaline
Honey

Oils
Acid
Nut oils
Butter
Cream

Alkaline
Olive oil
Soy
Sesame
Sunflower
Corn
Safflower
Cottonseed
Margarine

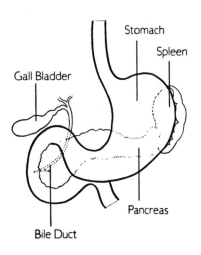

Stomach

Spleen

Gall Bladder

Pancreas

Bile Duct

"In the Five Element Theory, the spleen is located at the center; when the spleen is sick, the entire body is fundamentally sick. These days it is not rare for the spleen to be diseased. We eat too much sweet food."

NABORU MURAMOTO

Spleen and Pancreas

The spleen is the other organ for the Earth element. It stores blood and destroys old blood cells, and is the reserve organ for blood formation in the adult. In the fetus, however, it is an important organ for blood formation, especially red blood cells. The spleen also consists of lymphatic tissue and produces plasma cells, which make antibodies, tying the spleen to the immunologic system and thus, into protection against various diseases.

The pancreas is associated with the spleen as an Earth organ in Chinese medicine. It secretes hormones into the blood, regulating the body's use of glucose. Insulin, the pancreas' main hormone, lowers the blood sugar level by stimulating glucose use by the cells, or the pancreas may secrete the hormone glucagon into the blood, raising the blood sugar level. The other function of the pancreas is the secretion of pancreatic enzymes directly into the small intestine assisting in the digestion of fats, proteins, and carbohydrates.

The flavor of sweetness is associated with the Earth element and just as a little sweetness stimulates the spleen and pancreas, too much sweet food can injure them, and diminish your energy level. This suggests that a long-term effect of excessive use of sugar may overwork and thus weaken the pancreas, leading to insufficient insulin or a weak insulin response. This creates the inability to clear and use up the sugar in the blood, leading to "high blood sugar" known as diabetes. An over-response of the pancreas from sugar and food intake, putting out too much insulin is the mechanism involved in the problem called "hypoglycemia," or low blood sugar. So, watch out for that sweet tooth as it can put cavities in your teeth and decay your body as well as mess up your digestion.

The body makes its own sugar, "human glucose," the fuel on which the body runs, from all the foods you take in. Proteins in the form of amino acids, fats as fatty acids, and starches as simple and complex carbohydrates, can all be converted to glucose to run the body machine. When needed, there is also a reverse process when glucose is converted back, either to glycogen and stored in the liver, to amino acids for muscle storage, or to fatty acids to go into fatty tissue. An over-use (abuse) of sugar will produce mainly fat, first deposited in the most inactive areas, especially the abdomen, thighs, and buttocks; and then later, with chronic excess, in the internal organs, the blood vessels, heart, or kidneys. Conversely, a low sugar intake allows the body to change excess fats to glucose for ready use, clearing away those flabby hidden curves.

Centering

What does being centered mean, and how can we achieve this? Centering is grounding, or being in contact with the Earth. We exist as a medium between Heaven and Earth, of spirit and matter of which we consist. Centering also, as I see it, has to do with finding a balance in which we are aware of our polarities, the *yin* and *yang* qualities of Earth and Heaven, left and right, inner and outer.

Picture this center as a point within you that is the meeting point of a three-dimensional cross. The horizontal line extends left and right, connecting your two sides. This reflects the integration of the functions of the left and right brain hemispheres. Being centered involves an awareness of both the left brain's linear, sequential, logical, time-oriented and verbal functions, and the right brain's timeless, intuitive images existing in space. Our educational system stresses left brain development, but the quieting of this thinking side and the stimulus of right brain activity is correlated with relaxation, and relaxation is necessary for centering. Experiencing the arts of music, painting, or dance will stimulate right-brain awareness. Bringing your dreams from deep sleep into waking consciousness will also help.

Next, the vertical line of above/below is your mind and body. The mind contains your thinking and the body is your senses. Yet to experience your senses, information must be communicated to your brain. The mind and body can easily battle. The mind has the power to override the body to a certain extent, only to have the body express itself possibly in anger throughout its various parts, resulting in dis-ease. The balancing of these two poles is a key to long-range health.

The third line of your three-dimensional cross runs from inside to outside—in the center is you. The outer world, the environment of nature and other people, and the inner world of senses, feelings, thoughts, and inner voices must continually communicate. Through the center we integrate these worlds. The point at which these three lines of life experience cross is your center.

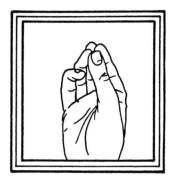

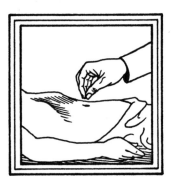

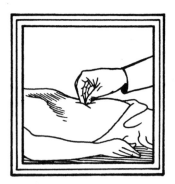

The way the Chinese evaluate the state of energy and balance (centeredness) in the body is by palpating the strength and position of the pulse at the navel, or umbilicus. That's the belly button, your first attachment to human life. Stand to the right side of a person lying flat on his/her back. Take the thumb and the first three fingers (leave out the pinky) of the right hand and hold the tips together firmly so that they look like a square. They should be touching. Place these three fingers and thumb over the navel so that the navel is centered between the fingers. Press gently, slowly, but firmly down until the pulse is felt. This is actually the abdominal aorta, the large blood vessel that goes from the heart into the legs. The pulse should beat strongly in the center. If not, it may be toward the left, right, upward, or downward. For example, a pulse that is felt above and to the right of the umbilicus might suggest that someone's energy is more focused to the active side (right) with the mind (upward part) playing a strong role.

Wherever the pulse is, you can help bring it toward the center by massaging gently for five minutes or so on the abdomen from the area where the pulse is toward the center of the umbilicus. This should help in centering someone's energy. If you have the opportunity, you can check it again later, or after a few days. Does it act similarly, or change? How does the pulse placement in your opinion relate to the person's energy state? You can likewise perform this exercise on yourself.

How else can you center yourself? Actually the question is how do you stay there (or get back there—as I believe this is your point of origin)? Your birth, actions, relationships, work, etc. take you on little journeys from this home, but you must always return to relax and replenish yourself. There are lots of ways to do this; some use "meditation," others "exercise," but really you, as an individual, must find your way each time from a multitude of possibilities.

One or many may work, and what works may change, as you do. That's nice, because it allows you to continue your life experiences. Don't get stuck in thinking you or anyone has "it." The ability to listen and see, to focus and adapt to that ever-changing moment of now is the key. This can be a formal practice which will help you open to your heart's wisdom, your mind's depth, and your body's senses, but it doesn't have to be. Just sitting or lying while relaxing and breathing deeply will be helpful. It could be dancing, walking, or running; being with a friend; making love; drawing a picture; listening to music; prayer; fantasy; focusing within or on an object; watching your thoughts; reading a book; doing your work; or really anything you enjoy as long as it helps you to let go of your tensions and resistances—and relax.

"Plenty is so little whilst we dance in the middle."

Arglsle

Late Summer Diet

Late summer is the beginning of harvest time. Fruits are falling ripe to the ground and vegetables are growing big and plump on the vines. Apples, grapes, tomatoes, beans, and zucchini are some of nature's gifts; squashes and pumpkins are still in preparation, the grain is close to harvest as well. Weather permitting, we may still eat as lightly as feels good, but as we come toward the autumn equinox, the cycle of darkness becomes dominant, and our balance shifts inward. This is a time when you can begin your building and toning program, which includes diet and exercise.

A building diet will give you a greater proportion of protein-rich foods; a little more fat than during spring and summer; and lots of good heating fuel from the whole grains. For vegetarians, whole grains with some beans can be the staple with lots of fresh and steamed vegetables. Some seeds and sprouts, nuts, beans, dairy products and eggs should also be included. If you don't eat dairy products and eggs, you can use more beans in the form of sprouts, cooked beans, or other products like tofu. Also, eating more seeds and nuts, or making seed or nut milks will help in building. Sesame tahini is a high-protein, high-calcium butter of sesame seeds that can be used as well in the diet. Meat eaters will have an easier time with this building diet, increasing their consumption of fish and poultry primarily, and adding only a little of the red meats. This diet can continue into autumn and winter to keep heat and strength together.

If you are doing this building diet, I recommend also taking a few days monthly, or seven days in the mid-autumn before it gets too cold, to do a juice cleanse to help eliminate the toxins that these richer, building foods also introduce. And to make it easy there are a great variety of fresh fruits and vegetables to make juice from at this time of year.

"Eat slowly; chew your food well and DON'T OVERLOAD. Eat only plain food, plenty of fresh vegetable matter, salads, ripe fruits. The richer foods, however, such as meats, eggs, starches, sweets, etc. should be taken more moderately and only in proportion to the work one does. In that way the food can be balanced properly and the digestion can go on more completely. Failure to live up to these simple, natural rules, will gradually lead to the operating table, but the operation will not remove the underlying cause and consequently will not bring the desired relief."

"Golden Rule of Health"
HERBS
Elaine Muhr

Exercise

These cleanses might be slightly less needed if you are also involved in a good exercise program that includes sweating, which helps elimination and cleansing of the body. A building exercise program could be working with weights, repetitive exercises like sit-ups, leg-lifts, or push-ups, as well as running, swimming, and other sports. As nature turns toward her inward cycle, so you may find yourself contracting, especially as it gets cold. Make sure to get a balance now and through autumn and winter of loosening and stretching exercises to help your body and joints stay loose and supple. Forward bends to touch the toes, backward arches, side to side stretches, and leg splits are all good.

If you go slowly and not beyond your limits, you'll see that the body will start stretching and opening up. It's important to keep muscles strong and relaxed to prevent pains and injury. Flexibility, endurance, and strength are a good combination and the outcome of a well-balanced exercise program.

Foods on Trial

There are three substances that are common to almost every American's diet, and a major reduction of these in your diet will improve your health and may even save your life. The three are refined sugar (sucrose), cow's milk, and alcohol. In my own experience, the elimination or great reduction of these substances has really changed positively the level of energy I experience and the way I feel. In moderation, anything can be handled, but certainly any major use of these substances, especially chronically, affects your health proportionately.

The Sugar Web

The sugar question is the major issue. Its hazards are generally not known by its users; in fact, most of our lives are filled with advertising in stores, television commercials, and magazines, for the use of refined sugar products, from breakfast cereals to soda pop to salad dressings. I believe that the broad use of refined sugar in our culture constitutes a major problem to the health of the people. Its high use, now over 100 pounds per person per year in the United States, is a primary source of illness, both physical and mental, affecting children and adults. It is the main contributor of the most common diseases known, tooth decay and obesity. Its omission, along with a limited intake of refined foods, and the free use of complex carbohydrates such as whole grains, is vital to food health.

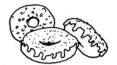

In his book, *Sugar Blues*, William Dufty makes a strong case for the elimination of refined sugar from out diet. He shares his own dramatic change for the good as he gave up sugar.

He looks at the history of sugar from the origin of refined sugar production, chronicling its use and the effects it has had on different societies. Countless examples of the introduction of refined sugar into a civilization show a rapid increase in infectious diseases and diabetes, and the decrease in the general level of health of those peoples. There are strong links between the sugar industry's beginnings and slavery in the 1600 and 1700s, and a well-studied correlation between the use of sugar-cured tobacco and lung cancer. (In naturally cured-dried tobacco, this is apparently not the case.)

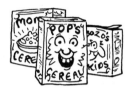

The physical ups and downs caused by sugar and the resulting mental imbalance, which include depression, anxiety, and irritability, may have created the need for the first mental institutions in France in the late 17th century. The brain cells are the most sensitive to changes in blood sugar levels. Sugar's degenerating effects can also be traced in certain situations when it was used as the main source of food. Medically, these mental extremes and physical degeneration may be understood when we look at sugar's depletion of many of the body's important nutrients such as protein, vitamin B, zinc, chromium, and manganese, all which are necessary for mental and emotional functioning, and whose deficiency has been associated with depression, fatigue, and low blood sugar.

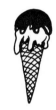

Refined sugar may also contribute to menstrual pain and problems in women, because of metabolic changes at that time. Elimination of sugar may help to remedy these menstrual problems. This makes sense in terms of the Chinese system as it correlates the health of the spleen with a balance of the sweet foods and menstrual regularity. An excess of sweet (sugar) may cause an imbalance in the spleen, which may, in turn, lead to menstrual difficulties.

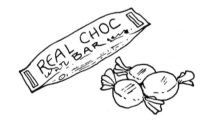

Actually, there are several kinds of sugars, all of which eventually get converted into glucose for the body's use. It is what is measured to determine "blood sugar." Glucose itself is usually found with other sugars in fruits and vegetables. The other sugars are: fructose (in fruit); maltose (in malt); lactose

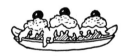

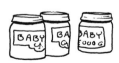

(in milk); date sugar; maple syrup; and honey, made from flower pollens by bees. I believe these sugars from whole foods, and those more simply extracted so they still contain a large amount of the initial food, do not overstimulate the pancreas or stress the hormonal system quite as much as refined sugars. Dextrose, a synthetic made from cornstarch, is the sugar constituent of a corn syrup.

Sucrose is refined sugar made from the sugar cane and the sugar beet, and has caloric energy, but no nutrition. The cane and beet are complete foods. However, in making "sugar," approximately 90 percent of the plant is removed. Molasses is the nutrient-rich syrup that is extracted to leave the crystal, which is then bleached to make "white sugar." This substance overstimulates the body and leaches nutrients from it. Light and brown sugars are refined white sugar with a little caramel added.

When you take refined sugar into your body, it is close to your own internally produced glucose and escapes digestive processing, passing right through the intestines to be absorbed rapidly into the blood, where the glucose level has been established in precise balance with oxygen. The glucose level rapidly rises, and the brain registers the imbalance, sending messages to the adrenals and the pancreas to pour out hormones (substances that are secreted *directly into the blood* affecting your metabolism).

Now the blood sugar level drops very fast as lots of sugar goes into the cells for use and we feel an "up," or rush of energy. But then the blood sugar drops too far (rebound effect); low blood sugar results and the next hormonal crisis ensues. Internal feedback stops the insulin output, and stimulates other adrenal and pancreatic hormones to raise the blood sugar to a homeostatic level. Your body and cells are saying, "We can't move, we want more sugar/energy," and you suffer a mini-withdrawal. This is the "down"—that tired feeling, slow brain, and the shakes, sweats, and nervousness, which occur while the body struggles to rebalance.

John W. Tintera, an endocrinologist, writes:

"It is quite possible to improve your disposition, increase your efficiency, and change your personality for the better. The way to do it is to avoid cane and beet sugars and all its forms and guises."

"After years of such days, the end result is damaged adrenals (our organs that are vital to life and help us deal with stress and crisis) *. . . When stress comes our way, we go to pieces, because we no longer have a healthy endocrine system to cope with it. Day to day efficiency lags, we're always tired, never seem to get anything done. We've got the Sugar Blues."*

SUGAR BLUES
William Dufty

Here's a 1912 quote from Dr. Robert Bresler, a New Jersey dentist, to tell us more:

Modern manufacturing of sugar has brought about entirely new diseases. The sugar of commerce is nothing else but concentrated crystallized acid. If, in former times sugar was so costly that only the wealthy could afford it, it was, from the natural economic standpoint, of no consequence. But, today, when because of its low cost, sugar has caused a degeneration of the people, it is time to insist on a general enlightenment.

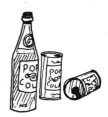

Alcohol, though dangerous, has not caused such widespread degeneration of a whole human race as sugar has, since it is not made of destructive acids. However, in England during the 1800s, sugar was used to speed up the fermenting process in the making of whiskey and ale. There was a huge outcry, with people claiming it made them sick and even hanging barkeeps for violating their "sacred drink."

Other examples and opinions about sugar include that of Sir Frederick Banting in 1929 in Panama, who noticed that plantation owners who ate large amounts of their refined sugar commonly had diabetes, while the cane cutters who ate only raw cane showed no diabetes. In the 1930s, a researching dentist, Dr. Weston Price, travelled the globe and described the destructive effect of refined foods and sugar on native populations in his book, *Nutrition and Physical Degeneration: A Comparison of Primitive and Modern Diets and Their Effect:*

People who live under so-called backward primitive conditions had excellent teeth and wonderful general health. They ate natural unrefined foods from their own locale. As soon as refined, sugared foods were imported, as a result of contact with civilization, physical degeneration began in a way that was definitely observable in a single generation.

Finally, here's a quote from *You Are All Sanpaku* written in 1964 by Sakurazana, a Japanese natural healer:

Western medicine and science has only begun to sound alarm signals over the fantastic increase in its per capita sugar consumption, in the United States especially. Their researchers and warnings are, I fear, many decades too late . . . I am confident that Western medicine will one day admit what has been known in the Orient for years; sugar is without question the number one murderer in the history of humanity . . .

If you are a sugar addict (sugar can be as physically addicting as a drug) these statements may inspire you to try eliminating sugar from your diet. See how you feel; I think you will find a surprising improvement.

I kicked the "sugar habit" several years ago. I experienced the loss of 40 to 50 pounds; a clear complexion finally at age 28; and the best, most consistent, and most productive energy I had ever known. The highs and lows of sugar going through my body disappeared, as well as the cravings for sugars and other substances. I enjoy food more, eat finer quality and tastier meals than ever before, and feel replenished after dinner rather than slow, groggy, and irritable. I wake up fresh and clear each morning, ready for the day.

Good alternatives for white sugar and other refined sweeteners include honey and pure maple syrup in small amounts. Honey is nutritious and can be used in recipes in place of sugar at about one-half to two-thirds the amounts as it is sweeter and more concentrated.

A fine substitute for chocolate is carob, also called "St. John's Bread." The carob pod grows on tall trees and has been known for thousands of years. This tasty and nutritional, large brown bean-like fruit can be eaten whole or ground in flour and used as a sweetener for cereal, milkshakes, or baking. Carob is six percent protein and 60 percent carbohydrate and contains calcium, phosphorous, and some iron. It can be used in digestive upsets and acts as a mild laxative.

Milk

Every American grows up thinking milk is one of nature's great offerings. And it is, when flowing from mother to child. But I'd like to say a few words about the overuse of cow's milk, and how it relates to our health and disease.

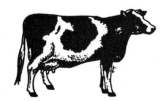

I was brought up with the idea that milk is the "perfect food" for everyone, and that all growing boys and girls should have three glasses of cold, pasteurized, homogenized milk a day. However, three to four colds per year were also considered normal. Neither idea is totally true! A fair trade for strong bones maybe, but there are lots of other sources of calcium and phosphorus. Recently, medical opinions reveal that cow's milk is for calves, and human mother's milk is for babies up to two or three, no older. This is the other extreme, and there must be a balance for each of us.

Many people can handle some cow's milk products, but goat's milk is even easier for humans to digest, as it is closer in composition to our mother's milk. Over half the people of the world find cow's milk indigestible: they don't have the proper enzymes in their bodies to process it. It seems true that the heated, pasteurized, homogenized, fortified-with-vitamins "milk" is indeed a culprit in causing congestive ailments ranging from the common cold to many chronic illnesses. I believe that any more than the moderate use of milk and its products in our diet is unhealthy.

Human milk has a much lower protein-to-carbohydrate ratio than cow's milk, two-and-one-half times less calcium, and has many antibodies to help fight infections. Cow's milk is a great building food, but it has its price. Glucose in excess gets stored as fatty acids in the abdomen, thighs, and buttocks, so that obesity may be closely related to the consumption of cow's milk with its high saturated fats and fatty acids, although sugars, cakes, and other treats also certainly play a role.

Usually, the positive side of this concentrated, "power" food is stressed rather than the difficulty of digestion and the problems of long-term or excessive use—it provides more than most bodies can handle. The caseinogen protein is hard for the adult human to digest. In fact, cow's milk is a common food allergy, even in babies under one year old who form antibodies against the large protein molecules of milk. Please realize that anything can be processed in small quantities by our marvelously resilient system, but that large amounts or long-term use of certain substances take their toll from the body.

Milk also has the effect on many people of causing a slowdown and dulling of their senses, as we see in the after-lunch nodding of school children after cookies and milk. It also may cause congestion of the mucous membranes, by thickening their secretions. The excess mucus can be the starting site for infections. Chronic indulgence in milk and its by-products, such as cheese, butter, cream, or yogurt is closely associated with atherosclerosis and I feel it may be a main cause of arthritic congestion and joint stiffness.

If you wish other high calcium foods as a substitute for milk, here are a few suggestion. Brazil nuts, almonds, and sesame seeds are very high in calcium. Highest in calcium per weight are the sea vegetables: kelp, dulse, Irish moss, and agar. Some greens, like collard, turnip, dandelion, and broccoli, are pretty good calcium foods.

It's very simple to make high-calcium nut milks in a blender with just nuts, water, a touch of honey or maple syrup, and a dash of sea salt. Almond, coconut, and cashew as well as sesame seeds all make good milks. Put one-half to one pound of almonds, coconut pieces, or shredded, unsweetened coconut into a blender. Cover with twice as much water. Add one tablespoon of honey or pure maple syrup, a dash of sea salt, and blend. Strain, keeping the liquid (nut milk), and re-use the nuts with the same amount of water again, and blend. Strain, once again and add the two liquids together. This is the nut milk! Drink as a tasty high-protein and high-calcium milky treat. Refrigerated, it will last a couple of days. However, it is best made fresh.

Alcohol

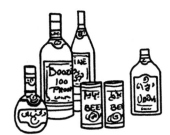

The third substance that needs no introduction but could be used less is alcohol (ethanol), which is rarely made very naturally these days. Even the potential nutrition of alcoholic drinks is "processed" away and some products have chemical additives. However, it still seems that small doses may be stimulating, helping the circulation, pinking up those cheeks, and actually the good quality stuff probably provides some nutrient content.

In excess, it still takes its toll. Physical aging, especially in the skin, face and eyes; liver disease; gastritis and bleeding problems; neuritis; and brain syndromes, are some of the resulting acute and chronic problems. In many county hospitals, people with diseases related to chronic ethanol abuse are responsible for a major part of the admissions. This problem is prevalent through all types of hospitals and all classes of people. Accidents are also common, "under the influence" of this dulling, inhibiting, central nervous system depressant.

Emotionally, its abuse is very handicapping. So, we need to keep our senses and remember, that even though a little drink may be relaxing and stimulate the circulation and appetite, too much can lead to lots of problems.

Herbs

Enough castigation of the American diet; let's be happy about all the good nourishing things around us. Getting back to the joys of Indian summer, and to the spleen, stomach, and the digestive system, there are a few herbs that will help the harmony of these areas.

Native American medicine is really the traditional American medicine and is very closely linked to Chinese medicine. They both have used herbal treatment in the context of an understanding of Heaven and Earth as a means of maintaining health.

Herbs have another close link—to present day pharmaceutical medicine. The human species has always used plants for healing. This seems to reflect an instinctive awareness of our bodies. Present-day science has allowed the active ingredients of herbs to be isolated, and with this knowledge, has been able both to extract the potent part of medicinal plants and to synthesize similar drugs with even stronger effects.

However, using whole herbs for many minor problems or to prevent illness may still be helpful. And they produce very few side effects.

For weak acidity, and to stimulate hydrochloric acid in the stomach for better digestion, make a mild tea from rosemary, dried orange peel, and/or ripe juniper berries, and drink a small cup one-half hour before meals. These herbs can be steeped by pouring boiling water over them, and letting them sit in a covered pot for 15–20 minutes. For weak digestion, avoid cold foods and drinking anything with your meals. Bitter foods, such as endive, dandelion greens, or chicory, will also help to strengthen the digestion.

For gas, indigestion, or hyperacidity, drink a seed tea like fennel, anise, fenugreek, or cardamom seed. These can be simmered in a closed pot for 15 minutes and then allowed to sit another 15 minutes before drinking. A few of these seeds, especially fennel or anise, can also be chewed as an after-meal digestive aid.

Licorice root (*Glycyrrhiza glabra*), named the "great peace-maker" by the Chinese, is a soothing herb for the digestive tract, a calming aid, and works as a mild laxative as well. Being gentle, it is a good herb for children too. It is also commonly used for sore throats, coughs, and colds. Licorice root, mixed with peppermint and fenugreek seeds, makes a nice after-dinner tea.

An herb that is also excellent to calm a nervous stomach is catnip (*Nepetu cataria*). Steep one teaspoon per cup for 20 minutes and drink warm. Some other stomach herbs are thyme, cinnamon, chamomile, ginseng, clove, and caraway.

For the health of the spleen, building immunity and increasing resistance to illness, try fresh romaine, parsley and/or celery juice, which also calms the nerves. Green juices, including comfrey leaf and wheatgrass, made fresh, are very energizing and healing. And if you're travelling, ripe juniper berries, 3 or 4 eaten several times a day, may be helpful for keeping up resistance to illness.

Two good herbs for general use and cleansing and toning the spleen are parsley and chamomile. Parsley leaf (*Petroselinum satiuum*), eaten fresh in salads, or steeped as tea, is a diuretic and expectorant, and helps cleanse the kidneys, spleen and intestines. It is also known to be effective for female problems; for gallstones, and for liver ailments. Parsley is high in potassium, iron, vitamins A and C, manganese, and copper. It is a good general herb and food and can be used freely. Steep a bunch in 2–3 cups of water and drink through the day.

A good herb for stomach and spleen is chamomile flowers. Chamomile (*Matricaria chamomilla*), is one of the old and very popular herbs. The German, or Hungarian, variety is most commonly used; it acts as a soothing relief for the stomach, stimulates the appetite, and helps in calming the nervous system.

Chamomile is used, too, in spleen problems and for menstrual irregularities as well as for hair rinses, in baths, and in skin lotions to keep the tissues and skin young and bright and to relieve weariness. It is especially good in a foot bath with peppermint. Chamomile tea is also strained to use as an eye wash to relieve tired or irritated eyes. It is considered effective for kidneys, bladder problems, colds, nervous disorders, and to help expel worms.

Other herbs for the spleen are fennel, golden seal, dandelion, white oak bark, and chicory.

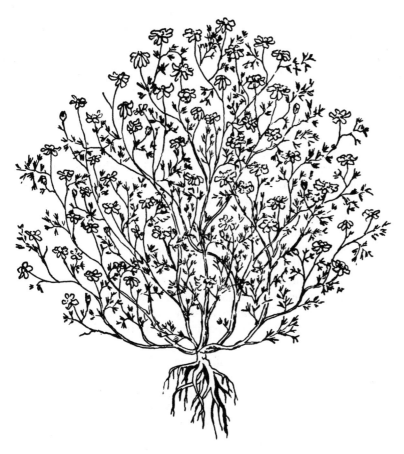

Chamomile
Matricaria chamomilla

Summary

The late, or Indian, summer is the time of transition in nature and of adjustment in our lives. It marks the shift from the outward expression of spring and summer to the inward focus of autumn and winter. This time is associated with the Earth element, which represents the stable center of our existence, fertile and focused on form and manifestation.

As we shift our lightness in diet toward a bit more density, giving us more fuel, we may feel stronger and more able to work. This building program may include heavier protein and fat foods, whole grains, seeds, nuts and beans. But remember, your diet has to always have a good percentage of fresh fruits and vegetables too, for a proper alkaline balance. It's a good time to work on your food-combining and eating habits.

You can start toning up in your exercise program as well to help build your strength. Working with weights, as well as calisthenics and isometrics, are good exercise programs to begin now, but you should keep your outdoor activities and sports going as long as possible too. This daily exercise will help regulate your weight and balance the tendency to gain a few pounds through the fall and winter.

The organs relating to this late summer time and the Earth element are the stomach and spleen. These two work together to digest your foods and distribute the resulting energy throughout the body. Nourishment is important to your energy state and well being, so the proper functioning of these two organs is vital to your feeling good and to preventing illness. Your eating habits are key to keeping your digestion working efficiently and maintaining a strong stomach and spleen.

Clarity in your diet will see you through many external problems and through seasonal transition. Your diet affects all aspects of your life—your work, productivity, personality, your sleep and dreams, how you feel from day to day, your health or illness, and where you live in your mind and on the earth. In the *Center* is where we go to have a look at life's show; all we have to do is flow—that's the real way to grow. So *let's go.*

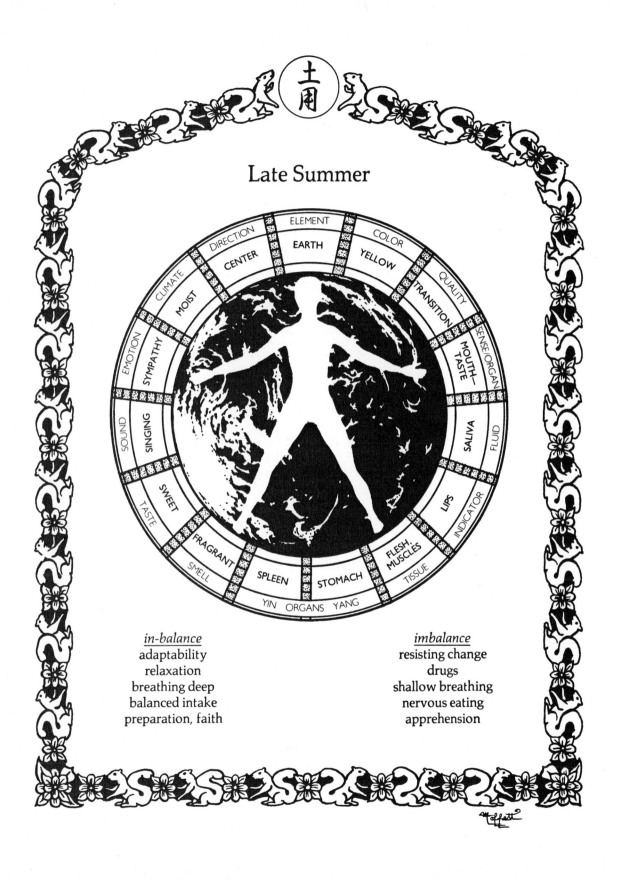

Late Summer

土用

ELEMENT — EARTH
DIRECTION — CENTER
COLOR — YELLOW
CLIMATE — MOIST
QUALITY — TRANSITION
EMOTION — SYMPATHY
SENSE/ORGAN — MOUTH-TASTE
SOUND — SINGING
FLUID — SALIVA
TASTE — SWEET
INDICATOR — LIPS
SMELL — FRAGRANT
YIN ORGANS — SPLEEN
YANG — STOMACH
TISSUE — FLESH, MUSCLES

in-balance
adaptability
relaxation
breathing deep
balanced intake
preparation, faith

imbalance
resisting change
drugs
shallow breathing
nervous eating
apprehension

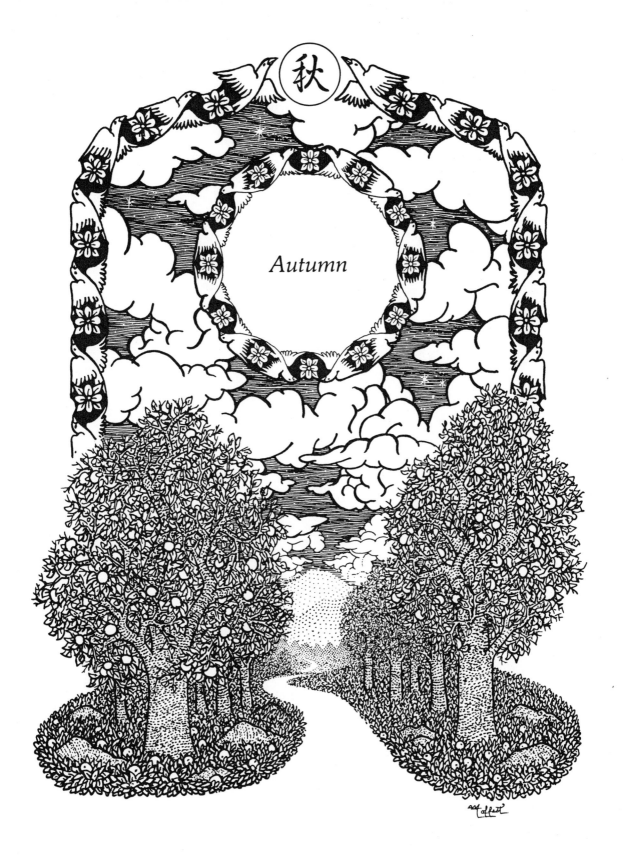

Autumn

Autumn Harvest

HELLO FRIENDS—WELCOME TO AUTUMN. This is the season of the harvest, the fruition of all the growth of spring and summer. This is true for us as well, as we receive the benefits from our work and projects, our relationships, and our health from all the energy we put into these areas during the last six months. The seeds we have sown, now shall we reap.

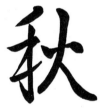

Autumn is the season of gathering nature's products before winter's rest. Fruits, vegetables, nuts, and grains are all abundant; for example, citrus fruits, grapes, apples, pears, tomatoes, walnuts, sunflower seeds, brown rice, corn, and wheat. As symbols of harvest and Halloween, squashes and pumpkins become plentiful by mid-autumn.

We store the excess for the long winter ahead. Canning extra fruits and vegetables, grain and seed storage, and obtaining our wood or fuel stock and warm clothing for the cold, darker months are important now. Even if we're not growing our own food, autumn is still a time of preparation for the season of rest.

Autumn also marks the beginning of a cycle of personal turning within; its first day, September 23rd, is the equinox day, when night's darkness finally equals the length of the day. After this, nights become longer than days, until the winter solstice, the longest night, on December 21st. In autumn, our time seems more directed toward our work, our families, and projects at home.

These days of seasonal change around the equinox are a perfect time to cleanse your body and lighten yourself for fall's work. Like early spring, early autumn is a good time for cleansing, but afterwards your diet may be fuller, richer, and more heat-producing than in spring, in order to carry you through the chill of late autumn and winter.

It's time to clear away finished projects and open up to the inner wisdom that you can experience in activities like contemplation, writing, reading, and nurturing your family as part of your preparation for the depths of winter. You will then feel a lot better and this potentially difficult transition will be easier.

Change is an inherent process in our lives and possibly the only "truth" in the universe. If you adapt yourself to the changes that come with the seasons, you will maintain health. You must gain control of your internal climates (emotions) and stay protected from the external climates. Maintaining a healthy state depends especially on a balance of outward activities and regular, inward-directed activities.

Through a daily discipline of inner attention and physical exercise, you can create a more open, resilient, and supple body; a mentally and physically relaxed state; and a stronger resistance to disease. Using your body in dancing, yoga, tai chi, jump rope, or other solo-exercises, and learning quiet breathing and relaxation will start your days in a more balanced, open state. And physical activity and exertion will help you relax more deeply and sleep more soundly.

Metal Element

Metal in the Chinese Five Element theory is associated with autumn, and represents the mineral ores and salts of the Earth. These function in creating structure and communication. For instance, metal wires establish connections and conduct electricity. Your brain and nervous system is really analogous to electrical wiring. Most forms of communication like the telephone, television, and transportation depend on this Metal element.

The Chinese do not include the element Air in their Five Element system, whereas several other systems do. This is often confusing, but the associations with Metal in the Chinese system are very similar to the aspects of Air in astrology, and in both Eastern Indian and North American Indian systems.

Both Air and Metal energies are expressed in the inner workings and activities of the mind, and in developing ideas, writing, and speaking. Degrees of mental clarity can be compared to Metal's varying forms, which range from crude, impure, and dense ore to a shining, crystal-clear gem.

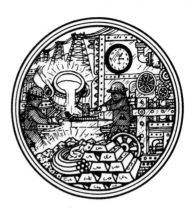

The Metal element is connected with many other outer and inner aspects. It is associated with the western direction, and with the color white. Whiteness in the facial hue may represent a Metal imbalance, mainly seen in the skin around the eyes and in the cheeks. This may be especially noticeable in someone who has had a bad cold, or acute or chronic lung problems, or in someone who has recently been experiencing great worry, grief, or sorrow, the emotions corresponding to the Metal element.

These feelings can be a healthy response, but if extreme or prolonged may injure the lungs or large intestine, which are the two body organs associated with the Metal element. Worry may cause poor, shallow breathing or the holding back of proper elimination, both important functions of the lungs and large intestine. Characteristic of Metal is the sound or expression of weeping or crying, which can be a good outlet for sorrow or grief.

Appropriately, the sense organ for the Metal element is the nose, and the associated sense is smell. The flavor corresponding to this element is the pungent or spicy one, as found in certain aromatic cheeses like Roquefort, Brie and Camembert, as well as peppers, mustard, and other spices. This flavor "opens up" the senses, clears the sinuses, and stimulates the lungs, but too much can also be injurious to the lungs. Often, a craving for spicy foods or a frank distaste for them may suggest an imbalance in the Metal element.

Metal's body fluid is mucus, and the climate is dryness. However, extreme dryness can injure this element, as can its opposite climate, dampness. On the one hand, being very attracted to dry weather, or on the other, intensely disliking dryness may suggest an imbalance in the Metal element.

The mucous membranes contain two types of cells: serous, producing a watery fluid, and mucous cells, which produce a thicker secretion. It is the mucus that protects and coats the mucous linings, while the serous fluid helps wash debris and bacteria, for example, from these sensitive membranes. Normally, there is a higher percentage of serous cells along these linings. Excessive mucus is actually a relative state of dryness from inadequate water intake, too much mucus-producing food, or from a Metal element imbalance. This increased mucus is a place of potential stagnation and thus a good growing medium for microorganisms. The association of the Metal imbalance with a runny nose, sinus congestion, coughs and the incidence of colds is important.

When a person whose Metal energy is imbalanced experiences excitement or other change, he or she will respond by coughing. Coughing expels mucus from the airway and the lungs, or can just cause more irritation in an already inflamed respiratory tract. On a symbolic level, coughing resists and attempts to expel anything not wanted: communication, emotions, or an unwelcome change.

Breathing involves both the intake of new air (energy) during inspiration, and the elimination of the old (that which is no longer needed) in expiration. These words, "inspire" and "expire," suggest a living and dying process and that's what breathing is truly about, from your first breath on arriving into Earth's atmosphere to your last one when you exit. The Buddhists see each inbreath as giving new life and each breath out as a little death. Thus, your deepest attitudes toward living and dying may affect your breathing process and the health of the Metal element in your body.

You can gloomily experience every breath or change in terms of what you're losing, focusing on what you will no longer have. Or you can be open and joyful, welcoming each breath and each change in your life by looking toward the new experience and growth it will bring. When you dwell on the melancholy, you are prone to injury of the Metal element and in turn to colds, lung ailments, and digestive problems.

Your bowel habits may reflect your approach to change; for instance, you may hold on to fecal matter until you even experience pain, or you can freely let go of your waste products. This "holding on" occurs not just in the rectum, but throughout the body, involving muscular tightness, mental tension, and other restrictions of bodily functions. You may need to re-train yourself to more easily and efficiently process your foods, thoughts, and emotions.

The tissues of the body governed by the Metal element are the skin and body hair. Thus, this element fortifies the skin and hair, and their health often reflects that of the lungs and large

"The lungs are the administrators responsible for orderly and lawful conduct."
CHINESE FOLK MEDICINE

"The lower intestines are like the officials who propagate the Right Way of Living and they generate evolution and change."
NEI CHING

intestine. In fact, the skin acts as the third lung, being the outer shell in contact with the air.

In both Chinese and Western medicine, lung and skin problems are seen as closely related. Asthma, eczema, and skin rashes are commonly associated with colds and lung infections. Dry or oily skin may also suggest an imbalance. Like the large intestine, the skin is important to elimination. The skin can help in getting rid of excess wastes. Acne sores and skin boils are common examples of this elimination, and can occur even more while one is on a juice cleanse.

The body hair, Metal's "indicator," is a more subtle diagnostic tool. I do not totally understand its association, nor have I been impressed with its clinical use. However, with attention to changes in the body hair and to the skin's health and vitality, we can get some reading on the state of well-being of the Metal element.

Lungs and Large Intestine

In the Chinese system, the Metal element is associated with the lungs and the large intestine, and the autumn season. This is a good time to work at keeping these organs strong and healthy. If you are one of those with a history of digestive or bowel weakness, or of long winters of colds and lung problems, this is the time to prepare yourself for staying well this fall and winter.

The lungs and the large intestine are two areas of your body that must stay clean for their best function, and often have difficulty when they are contaminated by the environmental pollutants of cities, by smoking habits, and by the dietary excesses common to the American culture. So, problems in these organs can be helped by first removing the harmful agents, and then cleansing the body. You may have to muster your willpower, but doing this will effect changes in your entire physical and mental state.

Our lungs communicate between the inner and outer atmospheres, and constitute a key organ for our existence. Performing the essential function of respiration, the lungs exchange oxygen and carbon dioxide through the pulmonary (lung) capillaries at the fine membranes where blood and air meet. We take in and use oxygen (O_2) and eliminate carbon dioxide (CO_2). As our ecological complements, plants breathe in CO_2

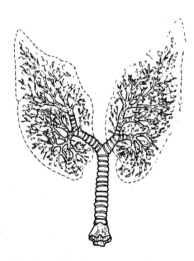

The lungs inhale oxygen and exhale carbon dioxide. Plants inhale carbon dioxide and exhale oxygen. The Bronchial Tree reflects the form of its partners in the full cycle of respiration

and expel O_2. Lung breathing is actually only the body's external respiration; internal respiration happens when each cell takes in oxygen brought by the blood circulation and expels carbon dioxide, which is then carried back to the lungs by the blood.

At rest, the average human breathes 12–15 times per minute. In deep relaxation this slows down, but with exercise, nervousness, or other increased oxygen need, the respiratory rate will increase.

Just as proper food is needed for energy and health, deep breathing and good air are vital to life. The fine membranes of the lungs were not really created to breathe smoke of any kind. We must do all we can to breathe the purest air—it still exists, though we may have to get feisty and ask our friends and our society not to pollute it.

Lungs do not like a cold, damp climate either, so keeping yourself warm and your chest, neck, head, and feet warm and dry may help you to prevent colds.

"The lungs are the rulers over autumn. Since the lungs correspond to the large intestine, both organs have to be treated together. The lungs are the stronghold and the root of the breath. Their condition manifests itself in the skin and body hair."

CHINESE FOLK MEDICINE

The large intestine is another important organ and, in our society, is one of the most overstressed ones. It is about five feet in length and travels around the edge of the abdomen. It is divided into the caecum, with the appendix attached; the ascending, transverse, descending, and sigmoid colons; and the rectum. Its main function is the absorption of water, but it also completes the absorption of nutrients such as sodium and other minerals, and houses friendly bacteria which help break down food and synthesize vitamins. This organ also forms, stores, and eliminates the feces.

The normal transit time, that is, the time it takes for food to pass from mouth to anus, is 24 to 36 hours, though some foods may either move faster or stay in the colon longer. A study of transit times and diets of many cultures shows that the naturalness of the diet and lifestyle may influence greatly the elimination time and the bulk of the feces. This in turn may affect the incidence of certain diseases such as diverticulitis and possibly even cancer of the colon.

Regular bowel movements occur naturally after eating a meal, since the gastrocolic reflex causes contraction of the rectum in response to distention of the stomach. This is true particularly in children, but as we get older, often the new conditioning of school and the stress of work affects this natural, lightening movement. Congesting diets high in meats,

Lungs and Large Intestine

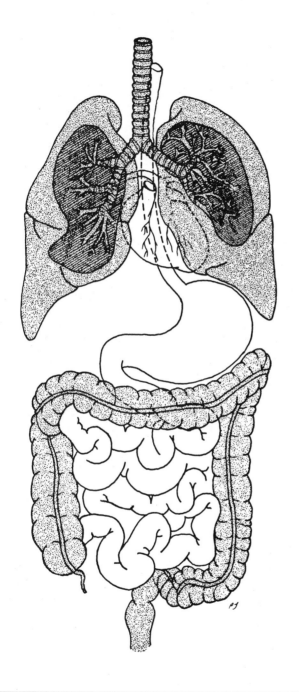

Lungs—the breath of life
Through their fine structure and large blood flow, the lungs act as mediators between air outside our bodies and the air within our blood stream.

Large Intestine—the fountain of youth
This organ deals primarily with the elimination of solid wastes from the body.

dairy, and refined foods, and poor eating habits, like eating on the run, also interfere with our regular bowel movements.

Congestion of the large intestine, both acute and chronic, often leads to the displacement and loss of tone of this organ and is the cause of many pains and illnesses. General abdominal discomfort and low and mid-backaches are often referred from the distention of the large intestine. In the Chinese system, the energy pathway, or meridian, for the large intestine includes the head, nose and sinuses, and neck. Pressure in the head and sinuses, headaches, sore throats, as well as crankiness, lack of energy, and even lack of enthusiasm for life, can thus come from a back-up in this organ.

Lung and Large Intestine Meridians

Lung—11 points
The lung meridian begins at the upper chest just below the clavicle and goes onto the arm, running along the thumb side of the palm surface of the arm and forearm. It continues over the pulse at the wrist and ends at the thumbnail.

Large Intestine—20 points
The large intestine meridian begins by the index fingernail, goes between the thumb and index finger, travels along the outside of the forearm and arm, onto the shoulder and the neck, then along the face and ends at the side of the nostril.

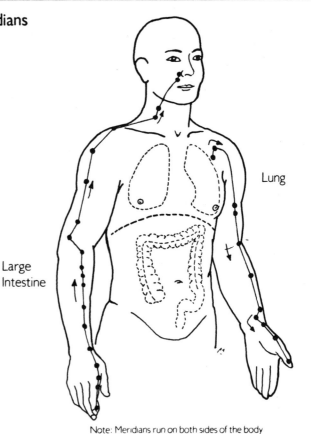

Lung

Large Intestine

Note: Meridians run on both sides of the body

The liver and gall bladder oversee the digestion of food and are important to the smooth function of the intestines. Dietary over-indulgences as well as the ingestion of poorly digestible substances such as alcohol, fatty foods, fried oils, and chemicals/preservatives are common and expected in our culture. These habits can create an overburdened, sluggish liver, causing slow intestinal functioning, and thus allow a buildup of even more toxins. This situation may then lead to problems like awakening congested in the morning, with sinus mucus, or with back stiffness, abdominal discomfort, or cramps, and it may be hard to get going for the day.

A diet high in natural foods—fresh fruits, raw or lightly steamed vegetables, and whole grains, will assist good elimination and keep the intestines well-toned. A low-fat diet, high in fiber foods (roughage) like greens and grains, is not only helpful for good elimination but may also help to prevent cancer of the colon.

The lungs have to do with balance in the body and seeing that justice exists among all the organs. The lungs are also the recipient of the Heavenly energy; with each "inspiration," we breathe in the pure spirit of Heaven.

The rhythm of the breath also governs the other rhythmic cycles in the body. Your breathing paces and keeps the heart rhythm and the blood circulation in order. The lungs also relate to the vital or instinctual energy, the basic life force, for respiration is essential to life.

The large intestine lets us know when we are in our "right way of living." Our ability to choose what we need for nourishment, to extract what we must use, and to eliminate wastes is important to grow properly, and to "generate evolution and change."

Colds

If your ability to handle and eliminate waste is weak, or if you take in more than you need, garbage may pile up inside the large intestine, to be dealt with by other areas of the body. The common cold is often experienced as an expression from the sinuses and lungs, but this problem is actually related to the large intestine and to poor elimination of wastes from the body.

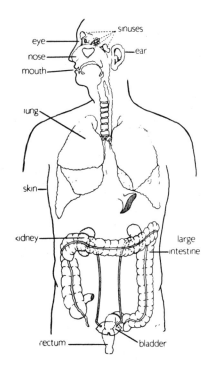

eye
nose
mouth
lung
skin
kidney
sinuses
ear
large
intestine
rectum
bladder

Elimination Organs

Primary
Large intestine
Kidneys
Lungs
Skin

Secondary
Sinuses
Sense Organs

The colon is one of the main organs of elimination, clearing toxins from the body helped by the lungs, kidneys, and skin. A slowing down of the intestines may result if the diet is high in unnatural, preserved, or processed foods; or high in mucus-forming foods such as meats, dairy products, sweets, and starches like bread and noodles; or if you are nervous or "up-tight." Then putrefaction and/or fermentation takes place, which creates even more toxicity in the system.

Mucus in the intestines not only leads to poor assimilation, but provides a site for bacteria and viruses to grow, just as it does in other parts of the body like the sinuses and respiratory tract. If your body cannot handle toxins through the normal eliminative systems, the excess toxins and mucus may begin pouring out through the sinuses. The pouring forth of mucus is in fact a cleansing as the body tries to get better; but full head, full mind, and no energy may be the result until this process completes itself. You can stimulate this cleansing process by drinking lots of fluids—water, juices, teas, and soups—and by getting proper rest and staying warm, rather than blocking elimination by taking cold tablets and eating congesting foods.

Unexpressed feelings and blocked creative energies also contribute to this head congestion and can weaken your physical resistance. Lower resistance allows cold viruses to move into your cells and multiply, creating that "flu-ey" feeling. This vulnerable state can also result from overwork, mental confusion and conflicts, inadequate sleep, and from emotional stress.

Illness will put you right where you need to be, lying quietly to let your head clear, and getting the rest and recharging that you need. The body treatment for colds is rest, fluids, sweats—in general, a cleansing and replenishing process to enhance elimination and gather new strength. Viruses cannot attack a healthy human organism. Often, getting in touch with your feelings and expressing them, or taking care of what you've been putting off, will also help the body cleansing process along.

The prevention and cure for the common cold is to stay in tune with your life and to develop common-sense attention to your diet, your physical activity, your emotional state, and to rest and relaxation. Learning to pace and nurture yourself and your loved ones is important.

Moderation is key to prevention of illness and to health

maintenance. A balance of intake of food and output of energy as work or exercise will affect your day-to-day health. Remember that extremes tend to create their opposites, as well. Excessive activity may require periods of prolonged rest, and fasting from food can lead to overeating. A new understanding of foods as energy, what they do, and how they affect you is very important. Learning to relax mentally and to express your emotions is vital to keeping your energy flowing.

Autumn Cleansing

A week or so of juice cleansing in early to mid-autumn will give you a boost of energy and may eliminate any potential illness you have stored away, either by flushing out excesses or by improving organ functions. There are, of course, lots of fruits and vegetables available for juicing at harvest time. The *Master Cleanser* is again a good choice; or apple-pear juice, orange juice, or other fruit juices in the morning, with vegetable juices like carrot, beet, celery, zucchini, or parsley in the afternoon and evening.

Since it is autumn, the grape harvest will be in, and this fruit is a fine cleanser, harmonizing the body and acting as a tonic for the lungs and large intestine. Five to seven days of freshly squeezed (you will need a juicer) grape juice will be a delightful autumn cleanse, or eating only grapes for a week will work wonders. You might drink a couple of glasses of lemonade each day to balance flavors if the grapes become too sweet. Taking one tablespoon of cold-pressed olive oil twice daily, as well as one cup of an herbal laxative tea on rising and before bed, will help keep the intestines moving.

It's good to dilute many juices with some water, and to drink them slowly, even chewing them a bit to allow the saliva's enzymatic action in your mouth. Your mouth and teeth are your "Number One" digestors, and those pearly whites and gums need regular care, especially during cleansing just as your tongue may as it gets more coated. Keep this area clean with regular brushing and flossing. Don't let yesterday's meals linger between teeth and gums; that's how decay happens.

During cleansing, you must be sure to bathe daily and brush your skin with a loofa sponge or skin brush to remove dead cells and to stimulate the clearing of toxins. Your skin's health is important to the lungs, and its regular care will help general

MOKU-YOKU SHIN-TAI
TOGAN   SHU-JO
SHIN-JIN   MU-KU
NAIGE- KO KETSU

from the wall at Tassajara,
Zen Mountain Center

As I bathe this body
I vow with all sentient beings
to wash from this body
and mind all dust
and confusion
and feel healthy and clean
within and without

elimination. Exercise, with a good sweat, is great to facilitate skin and body cleansing before you bathe.

At the end of a bath or shower, using cold water will close the skin pores and prevent heat loss and vulnerability to colds, as well as stimulate skin circulation. This is even more important as the weather gets colder because when going into a cold area after a hot bath or shower, your skin pores and body are open to a deeper penetration by the chill.

A nice replenishment for the hair and scalp is an overnight wheat germ oil treatment. Wheat germ oil is high in vitamin E and is very nourishing to the skin and hair. Before bed, apply freely to your hair and scalp, and massage. Wrap your head in a loose linen or towel. After rising in the morning, do a bit of exercise, then shampoo your hair.

Jojoba oil, extracted from the bean of a desert plant, is very rich in nutrients. It is specifically known to stimulate hair growth and nourish the hair and scalp. It may be used in place of the wheat germ oil.

Garlic

Another important lung aid that also facilitates cleansing and healing is garlic—a plant and herb, a food and medicine that has been used for centuries by many cultures. Also called "stinkweed" and the "poor man's medicine," garlic has been known to have healing powers as strong as its odor. It contains some protein, calcium, potassium, and phosphorus, plus vitamins B and C, but its main action lies in the allyl-sulphur bonds that release its strong sulphur odor and contribute to its germ-killing effect. Garlic acts medicinally as a stimulant, diuretic, diaphoretic, expectorant, antiseptic, disinfectant, and as a germicide and vermicide, meaning it kills germs and worms.

Garlic has also been said to ward off vampires and evil spirits. There are many stories, too, about how its use raw, or steeped in vinegar or in oil, has prevented the plague and other epidemic infections. Through the centuries people have treated colds, coughs, and sore throats with garlic, and used it for all kinds of lung ailments, including bronchitis, pneumonia, asthma, and tuberculosis.

Used internally it may be good for skin problems like boils and psoriasis, and externally it works as a disinfectant to

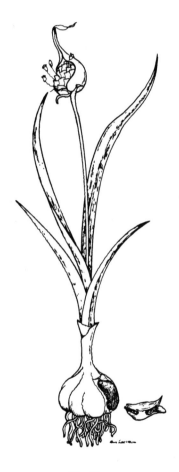

Garlic

wounds. However, do not apply garlic directly to the skin as it can cause blisters. Mashing some garlic with a little olive oil will make it more usable externally. During World War I in England, garlic-soaked bandages were applied to wounds to help prevent infection and promote healing.

Present-day uses for garlic include assisting the reduction of high blood pressure, as a treatment for worms, for colds, and other lung ailments. Used regularly in the diet, it may be indeed helpful in preventing colds, flus, and other infections. Try taking a couple of cloves a day, pressed into water or juice, or as garlic capsules, taking two twice daily. It is a good body cleanser, and a useful herbal preventive. Chewing parsley will help balance the strong breath odor. If you are not used to garlic, start with small amounts and develop a taste and smell for it. It is thought that your body begins to eliminate the garlic odor through the skin when you have had enough.

Garlic is easy to grow in the garden and is helpful as an insect repellent. It likes moist, sandy soil and good sun is important to its growth. An effective insect repellent is several cloves of garlic blended with water, strained through a cloth, and used as a spray for plants.

The odor and medicinal properties of garlic are in its essential oil. It is simple to extract this in olive oil; garlic oil then can be used for many purposes, from adding to salad dressing to rubbing on congested chests or even on the soles of the feet to prevent or remedy early colds.

Peel and chop enough cloves to fill half of a quart jar. Cover with good cold-pressed olive oil to about one inch above the garlic and place in a sunny window for five to seven days, shaking once a day. Then strain it well through a cheese cloth, and you have some strong-smelling garlic oil! The garlic that was soaking can be refrigerated and used in cooking, and the garlic oil will last months and can be used both internally and externally.

Colonics

High colonic irrigation, also called intestinal hydrotherapy, is a beneficial and non-toxic method of cleansing the large intestine with water. It has been used for thousands of years as a natural internal bath, long ago by entering a river or lake and using a hollow reed or bamboo tube to allow water to enter the rectum, and today by the fancy colonic machines with dials to regulate the pressure and temperature of the water. The Hindu scriptures write of the practice and benefits of enemas and colonics, and in 1500 B.C., the *Evers Papyrus*, a medical document, described its practice. Hippocrates, Galen, and Pare were all early advocates of enema therapy.

Many doctors have stated that constipation is one of the main causes of disease, and I feel that aging and death may well begin in the colon. To quote Dr. Ann Wigmore, founder of the Hippocrates Health Institute in Boston, in the *Naturama Health Care* paper, number 22:

"Hippocrates claimed that chronic disease came from auto-intoxication, i.e., self-poisoning due to constipation. The deposits of accumulated waste in the colon release toxins which inflame the nerves producing rheumatism, neuralgia, melancholia, hysteria, exzema, acne, headaches, and many many other health problems. Hippocrates also taught the way to handle disease—'Let Food Be Thy Medicine.' "

Colonic irrigations have been part of my own health program for several years, and after the initial weekly series, I took one monthly for a year and a half, and now use them seasonally. It is not a particularly uncomfortable experience, has basically no toxicity, and there are great benefits, particularly improving the tone of the large intestine.

The high colonic irrigation differs from an enema in that you rest comfortably on your back, while a short tube which has an inlet for water and an outlet for fecal matter is inserted into the lower rectum. This should all be regulated by an experienced therapist who can massage your abdomen and help you through the release of gas or any spasms. If you have any significant illness or specific colon problem, check with a doctor you trust who knows about colonics for referral to a trained colonic therapist.

You'll feel wonderful and much lighter afterward. Drink some orange juice, tea, or some potassium broth. Also, eating some liquid acidophilus or acidophilus yogurt, which contain live lactobacillus organisms, will help replace any lost colon bacteria. After a colonic you may feel a bit light-headed or weak temporarily. These feelings will pass after a short rest.

Such intestinal hydrotherapy has many benefits, and until we live purely it will be necessary and helpful. It helps relieve gas and spasms in the bowel, assists healing of digestive problems, and relieves many back and musculoskeletal pains, often caused by pressure from the intestines. Its greatest importance, however, is in eliminating toxins from the colon, in relieving stress on the liver, and in improving lymphatic and capillary function. Other added benefits may be improving the breath, clearing the skin, and enhancing the senses. When you begin to improve your diet with more natural and pesticide-free foods, and begin to eliminate toxins by cleansing and colonics, you will become younger, stronger, and more beautiful.

Your body is continually renewing itself, recreating its elements constantly. New blood cells are made daily and the total blood is replaced every 120 days, cells of the soft tissues are replaced every 12 weeks, and bone cells about every 12 months. The oldest cells in the body are supposedly no more than seven years old.

So, no matter how old you seem, you can be no older than seven! Isn't that a nice optimistic note?

Meditation

Since we are looking at the relationship of the Metal element and the mind in this section, it seems appropriate to discuss the practice of meditation; what it is; how to experience it; and some of its benefits, such as its potential to calm and clarify the mind.

Your mind has many dimensions with its ability to expand its attention; and to focus, limit, contain, and even close off that attention. Your mind is your body's transmitter and receiver. What is happening in your mind affects how you feel emotionally and physically. Ancient wisdom tells us, "As above, so below," and thus, what you are experiencing in your head influences your physical body, and vice versa, as your body state affects the working of your mind. I have pointed to this relationship in discussing both the breathing function of the lungs, and the elimination function of the large intestine: both breathing noxious gases and the state of constipation affect your mental capacities; likewise, your mental state can be reflected in the freedom of your bowels and in the ease of your breathing.

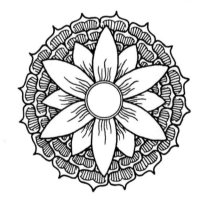

How you breathe determines how well you can center yourself, and thus relax. Just becoming aware of your breathing can help you realize and then clear body tensions and in turn open your mind to receive solutions to problems. Breathing is the basis of meditation.

There is much written on the subject of meditation, with such a multitude of definitions and practices that an attempt to comprehend this can be itself boggling to the mind. But I'll share my own experience of the process, and I hope it will inspire you to try to set aside the thinking mind for a while and experience a new openness to inner information. Scientists tell us that we use only a small percentage of our brain's potential, so we each must have a lot more to discover.

Meditation is a way of perceiving, of seeing. In a sense it puts you in a place that is almost separate from the mind, from which you can follow your mind's workings. Your awareness sits back and becomes just an onlooker to your mind and your life. Many describe it as a state in which nothing is going on. Our discussion of the brain in "Basics," described this human computer as having two primary functions, thinking and sensing, which empirically relate to left and right brain hemispheric functions respectively.

This bimodal character of the brain is crucial to how we experience life, also to the practice of meditation. One mode is active, thinking, time-oriented, and attempts to organize and manipulate our world. The other is receptive, sensing, timeless, and perceives and understands our external and internal environment without judgment.

In our technological, manipulative, and hyperactive culture, meditation has the effect of drawing energy from the thinking mode into the receptive, perceptive one. This may seem threatening since it sets aside our conditioning to be goal-oriented at all times and reverses our standard educational and work models. But by expanding your awareness to other areas of your brain, you allow a certain kind of knowledge to come to you which could not be obtained through the usual active mode.

Meditation moves you to a new balance, which is neither active or receptive, taking you to the center to experience both these realms. In Zen meditation, there is "sitting and being," allowing only the experience of the breath in the moment to be the focus. No other goals are sought, for this would lead to a focus on time passing, and create internal action. Both the seeking of pleasure and the avoidance of pain are suspended for the moment, and all attention is given to watching the breath ebb and flow.

Meditation has been practiced over the centuries to enhance sensory awareness and to alter perception of the environment and oneself. It is important to staying healthy as it facilitates a greater communication between our inner and outer worlds, and allows a deep state of rest and rejuvenation. Physiologically, meditation lowers the respiratory rate, increases the frequency of *alpha* brain waves, and facilitates muscular relaxation.

The effects of Transcendental Meditation (TM) in particular have been studied extensively. Testing shows that meditators experience an increased sense of intelligence (by psychological testing) and learning ability (recall testing); better performance (increased grade-point average) in school; faster reaction time; increased productivity and improved job performance and satisfaction with work; as well as better relationships at work. Physically TM helps the reduction of stress, possibly by lowering blood lactate levels; helps reduce insomnia; slows the heart rate; and normalizes blood pressure. It also helps regular meditators achieve a sense of greater adaptability and stability. Creativity as shown by the Torrence Creativity Test and personality development (Personality Orientation Index) seem enhanced too. Basically, meditation places you (your body and brain) into a resting state, *alpha*, wherein you can receive all kinds of new information and perspectives on things.

Meditation is not a goal but a process, a kind of awareness that is not alien to you, but is inherent in your nature. It is not something you have to *try* to do, but rather a process you must *allow* to happen, with as few preconceptions as possible. It is not someplace to go; it is a state of being.

You must merely give yourself the time for the experience. I find that the early morning is the best time, bringing clarity and energy to my day. Later on is also fine, but avoid meditating on a full stomach. It's better to wait for three hours after eating. Thus, before dinner or before sleep may be good times for you. You can sit on the floor, a pillow, or a chair, but don't lie down; keep this latter position for rest and sleep.

As busy as we all are, we can usually set aside 15 to 30

Look
When forsook
Close yer eyes
Take a look—

Arglsle

minutes once or twice a day for quiet conscious relaxation and clearing our minds of old and congested thoughts. You may see that many things you think you need to do are unnecessary, and those you really need to accomplish often take care of themselves. You may learn how to guide your energies rather than being controlled by your impulses. Sadly, we have been conditioned to live in the world outside of ourselves and create vast estates there while living in barren wastelands within. This will never create happiness.

Meditation practices take two primary paths. One is the focusing, or comtemplative, process in which you breathe, relax, and focus on your breath, a sound, a word ("mantra"), a picture, a candle, or some inner image. The other is the free-floating form where you sit and breathe and just watch what goes on without trying to manipulate at all.

Often exercise facilitates the meditative state. Yoga and tai chi chuan are examples, but nowadays runners and many devoted athletes are describing deep and profound experiences during and after exercise.

Breathing lays the groundwork for many meditation forms. Sit, relax, close your eyes, and breathe. You can formalize this by breathing in for seven counts (some use seven heartbeats), holding seven, then breathing out for seven. You may start with shorter holds, but as you relax, this breathing pattern will become easier. Breathe gently in through your nose and let it flow out through your mouth. Some practices have you breathe in and out through the nose. Do this for a few minutes and you will get used to this regular breathing pattern. Then just sit back and observe, watch your mind. Consider your thoughts as clouds floating by in an open blue sky. Do not get into them, just watch. If you get carried away, come back to your breath focus and counting.

Another exercise which is useful throughout the day, is to sit down and be with your awareness of the present moment. What is happening right now? No past or future, it is all happening in the present. This is a good one to take out in the world. You may become more aware of when you are worried, upset, or caught in thoughts of what you could or should have done or what someone did to you; or when you are feeling insecure or projecting your needs into future ideas and plans.

This kind of awareness is an important step toward finding

peace and joy in the world of now. You will eventually be able to incorporate this continual "meditation in motion," into all aspects of your life.

How and what you think affects everything around you and your experience of the world. The pollution on the planet earth reaches to the air, the water, the soil, and our food. But beyond this, there is mind pollution. If you buy into the media's picture of destruction and war, for example, this becomes the limit of your inner experience. That war, starvation, and destruction are inevitable is not true; they are based on the imbalance of the active, manipulating mode involving power, greed, fear, and a mental model of the world in which individual human life is seen as less important than the ideal of an individual's or country's lifestyle or belief system.

I believe that what we each think about definitely affects the collective consciousness. Rather than feeling helpless with personal or world difficulties you may sense that your thoughts have the power to change the world. Maharishi Mahesh Yogi, the first Western teacher of TM, has said that if we ever get one to two percent of the world population meditating, we will have world peace. Now that is powerful energy!

"Meditation is an empowering experience. In the stead of the narrow path of the outer-mind journey, with its many endless circles and its culs-de-sac, meditation is a journey to the everywhere of the universe, to the nowhere of the infinitesimal point at the center of the individual consciousness, as it joins the everywhere and the nowhere demonstrating they both are one."

JOY'S WAY
Brugh Joy, M.D.

Drugs

Meditation is a natural process which alters your state of awareness, by changing the focus from the active to the receptive mode. The more common way to accomplish this in our impatient society is through the use of drugs. Substances, both naturally occurring and laboratory synthesized, are used daily to alter physical and mental energy and the psyche. Drugs are an easy way into the receptive mode, and the meditative state is often simulated with alcohol, sedatives and tranquilizers, marijuana, and "psychedelic" drugs like psilocybin, mescaline, and lysergic acid-diethylamine (LSD).

The abuse of these and other drugs can be dangerous, but their use has helped in treatment of certain difficulties and has also allowed people to experience changes in their awareness which they then try to re-experience without drugs. I see this as a transition in a small part of the American culture during the 1960s and '70s. Now people are seeking this understanding in a more natural way, through learning to maintain a balance of the active and receptive modes from moment to moment.

Let's face it though, most of us still live in a drug-oriented society. Many drugs are used to treat illness, but many also help create "iatrogenic" (treatment-caused) illnesses. Children grow up watching their parents' pattern in both the social use of drugs and the use of prescribed and over-the-counter medicines as a first choice to treating any symptom or illness. The use of drugs as medicines is part of the same picture as using drugs to alter our psychological state.

It is time to break these patterns. Understanding your natural cycles will help you see the importance of creating healthier bodies by the use of good foods, exercise, and eliminating toxins in your life. Pleasure drugs are a lazy way to alter and control your energy. And the body will not be able to re-experience this relaxed or stimulated state without drugs unless you take the time to tune your machine to its most healthful state. As you become more concerned about every kind of substance you take into your body, you are increasingly learning to stay away from strong synthetic medicines as a first choice to cure your ills, and consider using more natural remedies.

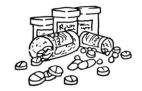

Some common drugs used to manipulate our energy state are caffeine, nicotine, sugar, alcohol, and marijuana, and tranquilizers Librium and Valium. Less prevalent are stimulants like cocaine and amphetamines; sedative-hypnotics like the barbiturates or opiates which include codeine, opium, morphine, heroin, and methadone; and the psychoactive class such as peyote (mescaline) cactus, psilocybin mushrooms and LSD. Some of these drugs are freely available in our grocery stores and pharmacies; some are found in nature; and others must be synthesized and illegally sold through a procurer and seller (a dealer). They all, however, have some degree of addiction, both physical and psychological.

The most common addictive drug, widely used in the entire food industry, and thus affecting everyone, is refined white sugar. The sugar habit is really one of the more difficult ones to kick.

Caffeine, a xanthine drug like aminophylline and theophylline which are used for asthma, occurs in such beverages as coffee, tea, cocoa, and "cola" soft drinks. Besides being a central nervous system and respiratory stimulant, which creates an "up" feeling, caffeine also stimulates smooth muscle activity, causing the bowels to move; dilates the bronchial tubes;

and stimulates the heart. It is metabolized by the liver and excreted through the kidneys. However, it also acts like a whip, stimulating the liver's use of its stored energy, and eventually depleting it. As the liver is your source of get-up-and-go power, caffeine is used a lot as a morning stimulant. It may be safer than other stimulants but eventually caffeine lowers your natural stores of energy and affects the health of the liver.

Other stimulants like cocaine and the amphetamines are very toxic to the body and wear it out rapidly. In medical school I was told that the average life span of a cocaine addict was 45 years, as it degenerates the body rapidly. While South American natives chew the whole coca leaves, the effect of this seems to be different from that of using the active crystals, extracted and "cut" with other substances as in North American "cocaine." I'll say simply, beware of this pleasure drug. Your whole body will appreciate your abstinence.

Amphetamines, sometimes used as "diet pills," seem to be passing out of vogue with the growing realization that their use really weakens people. The statement "speed kills" has a biological basis. Willpower and dietary changes, though slower to take effect, work much better than any of these drugs for weight loss.

Cigarette habits are an important drug use, too. Besides nicotine's immediate and multiple actions on the heart and blood vessels, and its irritating effect on the mucous membranes, bronchial tubes, and lungs, chronic cigarette smoking is clearly correlated with heart and blood vessel disease, and with cancer of the lungs.

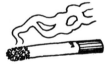

My own feeling is that smoking also acts psychologically to block communication between people. It's a defense—surrounded by a smoke screen, one avoids getting too close to others. It also interferes with other people's need to breathe clean air. This is a difficult addiction to stop, but it certainly is worth a try—in fact, as many tries as necessary to give it up for good.

Librium and Valium are the most widely prescribed drugs in the United States. This is probably true because doctors do not have the time to deal with the prevalent mental and emotional problems of their patients, and most of us as patients are too lazy to take the time or responsibility, or make the needed changes which will alleviate stress and conflict.

Librium and Valium, the "diazepams," have a subtle and

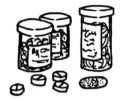

still unknown affect on the nervous system and general state of being. They, however, interfere with normal sleep by reducing the dream (REM) sleep. I feel that these drugs also interfere with creativity and give the user and his or her doctor a false sense of relief.

Our deeper disharmonies are not adequately treated merely by pacifying our outward tensions. We must bring our conflicts to the surface and resolve them.

The sedative-hypnotic and central nervous system depressant drugs like alcohol, barbiturates, and opiate-narcotics slow things down, create a sense of relaxation, and are primarily used by people to suppress emotional difficulties. Long-term alcohol use has many destructive effects. And while the barbiturates and opiates are not immediately toxic and have some clear-cut medicinal uses as with epilepsy, insomnia and pain, their long-term use creates emotional handicaps, as well as causing a slow-motion, detached character. The greatest danger lies in the physical and respiratory depressant effect that can cause death.

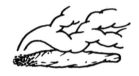

Marijuana (*Cannabis sativa* and *Cannabis indica*), a traditional medicinal herb, has become very prevalent as a pleasure drug throughout society. When the leaves and flower tops are smoked, it provides an euphoric effect, and switches on the sensing, receptive mode. While it doesn't seem to be particularly toxic, the lungs and bronchi suffer irritation which can lead to the "cannabis cough," and we don't really know its long-term effects. While there is no evidence that it causes chromosomal damage or sterility, it does seem to weaken the liver and possibly lowers resistance to illness. (Anything used habitually can become a crutch and can interfere with our state of clarity and our personal evolution as adults.)

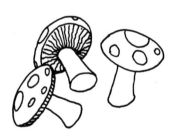

Psychoactive, or "psychedelic" drugs, act potently to change one's perception of reality. They may even simulate psychotic episodes. Both the psilocybin mushroom and the peyote (mescaline) cactus occur naturally, while LSD is made in the laboratory. The first two have been used in tribal and religious ceremonies, and their contemporary Western use as well as that of LSD seems to be affecting people's interests and lifestyles. These drugs both enhance the receptive mode and increase sensory awareness, decreasing focus on goal-oriented action, and diminishing boundaries as self and environment seem to blend, giving a sense that all is one. Although some of these effects may appear very much like the positive outcome of meditation, their use is in fact very draining to the user's system. Long-term use creates a physical wasting and a fragile psychological state.

Drugs often appear to have a beneficial short-term effect. Stimulants may temporarily help someone who is tired or who has low energy, while sedatives may aid the high-strung or stressed individual, but I feel that drugs are rarely a good answer. They all affect your physical, mental, and emotional states. Short-term use may lead to weakened resistance to illness and make you more vulnerable to colds, flus, hepatitis, lung and skin problems, while long-range effects help create many of the degenerating and chronic diseases through toxin buildup in the body, and by weakening specific organs and systems. Also, drug use may affect your mental and emotional stability. You must be careful about what you ingest and imbibe; a quest for immediate sensation and change may leave you in a place from which you may have a hard time getting back to a road where the sun shines and nature grows and flourishes.

"Let go of the old world and the new one will grow around you like a new skin."

DAS ENERGI
Paul Williams

Autumn Diet

If you have certain habits or addictions which you wish to clear out of your life, changing other aspects of your life, such as diet, exercise, even attitudes, can be very helpful. Often the added willpower and strength that comes from beginning new patterns affects positively those old habits. Just seeing yourself differently, without a cigarette or involved in a new situation, is very important in helping to change old habits.

It is good to begin autumn with a week's cleansing diet, of fruit and vegetable juices, or a grape fast. In general, however, the autumn diet is based on the building principle from Late Summer. For the omnivores, this includes more meats and dairy products, while the vegetarians will eat lots of grains and some nuts, beans, and seeds as well as more dairy and eggs if used. As you eat less and less fruit now, you can turn to more vegetables as well as grains, especially as the weather grows colder.

You may stay healthy by becoming aware of the complex effects of foods, watching and learning how they act in your body. The quantity and ratio of foods in your diet are important. For instance, a diet of primarily bread and cheese, both body congestors, will not keep you or your intestines free-flowing. Meats are concentrated energy, not particularly easy to assimilate, and they create more density and body heat than fruits and vegetables. Eating a lot of congesting foods, or simply overeating, tends to keep your internal state at the level of physical sensations and indulgences.

You should be aware that fruits and vegetables are body cleansers in general, but that bananas have a congesting effect while avocados and mushrooms act more as builders. The principal body builders are meats, fish, dairy products, nuts, beans, seeds, and grains in that order, but remember that these foods also create varying degrees of congestion. Other body congestors are noodles, potatoes, bread, cake, cookies, and all white flour, sugar, and chemical products.

Whole grains are high in vitamin B, and their cellulose content helps your intestines by stimulating good elimination. A diet consisting mainly of body cleansers along with whole grains, some building foods, and a limited intake of congestors will keep you clear, strong, and well. Lubricators include olive, sesame, and sunflower seed oil, margarine and butter, and some of these foods are needed to keep everything moving.

Diets are totally individual and related to your character, your activity, and to the climate in which you live. Since foods affect your energy level and your state of wellness, you can each choose by your diets and your life experiences how you wish to live.

Baked squash or pumpkin stuffed with a combination of brown and wild rice, sliced almonds, and mushrooms, is a great autumn dish.

Crisp autumn weather is a good time for soup. Vegetable-barley soup is a great treat and will keep you warm all over. Add some root vegetables like carrot, turnip, onion and garlic to the soaking barley, and simmer. Some greens like celery, comfrey, dandelion, kale, watercress, or spinach can be added at the end of cooking. Let them steep. Sea vegetables like dulse, kelp, or nori seaweed, as well as barley-miso-paste can be used to flavor the broth. Seasoning like rosemary, cayenne, ginger, or your own favorites will give that special touch.

Try making pumpkin or squash soup. And don't forget to bake the pumpkin seeds from your friendly jack-o'-lantern. These are really good for the intestines and are one of the foods used for treatment of worms.

Exercise

The autumn brings many sports such as football, soccer, basketball, as well as prepares you for the winter's fun of skiing, ice hockey, and snowmen. But in general, you might seem to be turning inwards, growing more *yin*, contracting; and you may need to concentrate more on staying loose and relaxed. Stretching, calisthenics, running, and hiking will all help. A strengthening program using weights and isometric exercises will build more muscles from your higher protein meals. Exercise keeps your weight in balance too, with the heavier autumn diet. It is natural to gain a few pounds during autumn and winter, so turn some of it into muscle as well as a little fat to keep you warmer.

Herbs

As autumn moves along, the energy in nature's plants starts going toward the roots. Leaves fall, and the life force goes within. As we too start feeling less active, we turn to the root herbs. Two roots that are common and very effective for the lungs and skin are burdock root and comfrey root. To extract their deeper essence, roots usually need to be simmered 20–30 minutes before drinking or steeping with leaf herbs.

Burdock root (*Arctium lappa*) is a tonic, diuretic, and an alterative. It has been used in chronic skin disorders like eczema and acne, as well as for boils and for lung ailments.

Comfrey (*Symphytum officinale*), both root and leaf, is known as one of the great healing plants. High in protein, vitamins, and minerals, it is a soothing expectorant, and a nutrient that aids cell growth, and is very healing to body tissues and bones as well as cleansing to wounds. Powdered comfrey root, ground up and applied as a poultice, stops bleeding. I have seen this occur several times when used on wounds and bleeding gums. The fresh leaf is used effectively for sprains and other injuries. Use cold or ice initially to reduce any swelling, then wrap a couple of comfrey leaves around an injury, cover with a moist hot cloth and wrap. Of course if an injury produces marked or prolonged pain or swelling, see a doctor. The root, taken daily as a tea, is also a tonic to the intestinal linings, mucous membranes, and the lungs.

Coltsfoot leaf acts as a lung tonic, too. But all tonic herbs work as slow builders when used daily (one teaspoon per cup,

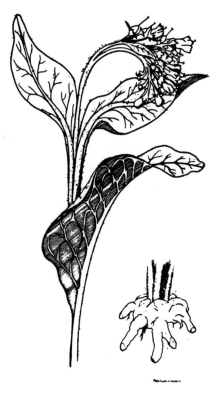

Comfrey
Symphytum officinale

149

twice daily) over a one to three month period. Some other lung herbs and expectorants are: licorice root, wild cherry bark, slippery elm, mullein, yerba santa, horehound, and Irish moss, a seaweed.

For more body heat and clearer lungs, ginger root, sliced and simmered 15–20 minutes then mixed with other herbs, is a great daily stimulant. Also a cloth or towel soaked in warm ginger root tea and applied to congested or cold areas can be very helpful to circulation. Cayenne pepper in your diet and in your socks may help keep you warm to well-done, stimulated, and with dancing, hot feet!

Many herbs tone the large intestine and give it a little nudge. One is cascara sagrada (*Rhamnus purshiana*), meaning "sacred bark," a bitter but effective laxative and tonic. Licorice root, sometimes called "sweetwood," is a gentle laxative, good for children. Oregon grape root is a little stronger and a good general tonic and laxative.

Dr. Christopher's "lower bowel tonic" is an effective combination of eight herbs to enhance elimination and tone the bowels, and contains: barberry bark, cascara sagrada bark, cayenne pepper, ginger root, golden seal root, lobelia leaf, raspberry leaves, and turkey rhubarb root, all ground together. Two capsules taken three times daily for a few months are helpful in healing bowel problems. Taper off then and experiment with foods which regulate bowel activity, such as whole grains, fruits, or vegetable roughage.

Summary

Autumn begins the dark, *yin* cycle, when the daylight lasts less than twelve hours. This is apparent after the autumn equinox, and peaks at the winter solstice. This *yin* cycle lasts until the spring equinox, when day and night are again equal. Autumn days bring inspirational ideas, school activities, and an increasing awareness of inner processes. Now is a good time for finishing projects begun in spring and summer, and beginning more inward and home-oriented projects. Autumn is the period of preparation for winter's resting time until the rebirth of spring.

In the Chinese system, the autumn season is governed by the energy of the Metal element, which is associated with communication and the workings of the mind. Mental well-being involves a positive self-image and being happy. You can accomplish this by taking responsibility for your happiness, by caring well for yourself and others, and by doing what gives you inward satisfaction and is also beneficial for your environment. It is true that no one else really makes you happy, it must come from within yourself; but those around you can definitely support your happiness. By being in touch with your feelings and sharing them with others, you will lose the sense of loneliness or separateness and begin to experience the connectedness of all things.

Clear thinking, openness to new ideas, and the ability to relax are all important mental virtues to cultivate. You may accomplish these by allowing yourself to experience the quiet, directed mind that has evolved in the Eastern cultures through centuries of meditation. By this practice of turning off the thinking mind—just being—you can balance yourself and be aware of both the conscious, rational thought, directed toward the outside world (active mode) and the creative, space-oriented (all is one), visual perceptions of the inner world (receptive mode).

The Metal element rules the organs of large intestine and lungs. The balance of intake, through breathing air and eating food, and output, breathing out, activity, and elimination, is crucial to staying healthy. The lungs are vulnerable to cold and damp climates, which can set the scene for colds and lung infections. The nose is the opening to the lungs and is in turn the sense organ for the Metal element, smell being the associated sense.

Keeping the nose and sinuses clean by occasional cleansing with salt water may help rid excess mucus. A teaspoon of sea salt to a pint of water can be used specifically for mucus problems by gargling and by breathing some into the nostrils and blowing the nose. You can do this same thing with plain water in the morning while showering or washing your face.

If you do get a cold or lung problem, you need to rest and drink lots of fluids; citrus juices are especially good for fever. Drinking herbal teas, soaking in a hot foot bath, or having a warm herbal enema or colonic irrigation all may be helpful. Dietary changes will help too, in preventing future health problems.

Constipation is a very common problem and often goes along with colds and lung problems. The major cause, though,

". . . the necessity of seeking within ourselves those defects we possess which cause us to work against Unity and out of harmony with the dictates of the Soul, and of eliminating these faults by developing the opposing virtues. . . . an honest self examination will disclose to us the nature of our errors. Our spiritual advisors, true physicians and intimate friends should all be able to assist us to obtain a faithful picture of ourselves, but the perfect method of learning this is by calm thought and meditation, and by bringing ourselves to such an atmosphere of peace that our Souls are able to speak to us through our conscience and intuition, and to guide us according to their wishes. If we can only set aside a short time every day, quite alone and in as quiet a place as possible, free from interruption, and merely sit or lie quietly, either keeping the mind a blank or calmly thinking of one's work in life, it will be found after a time that we get great help at such moments and, as it were, flashes of knowledge and guidance will be given to us."

HEAL THYSELF
Edward Bach

is the wrong diet. Eating devitalized foods, or too much meat or other congesting foods; or too much food at one time; or not eating roughage; or the side-effects of drugs; are all factors in constipation. Constipation can create a backup of toxicity through the body, and affect the muscular or nervous systems, creating tensions and exhaustion.

Poor intestinal elimination may affect the skin, another area of the body governed by the Metal element. In fact, you can look at the health of the skin to judge the health of this element.

An early autumn cleanse will help regulate the diet and provide enhanced elimination clearing the body of potential illness. The *Nei Ching* says, "The lower intestines are like the officials who propagate the right way of living, and they generate evolution and change." This is very important.

Eating and living habits are crucial to your well-being and important for your growth. It is time to assume total responsibility for how you feel on a day-to-day basis. Health begins with becoming aware of your energy and its balance—what you take in and what you put out. What's important is learning to listen to yourself from the inside so you do not have to become ill to change your life. Keeping your body and mind open and clear makes the way for positive thoughts and visions, and the *love from your heart* will fill every part.

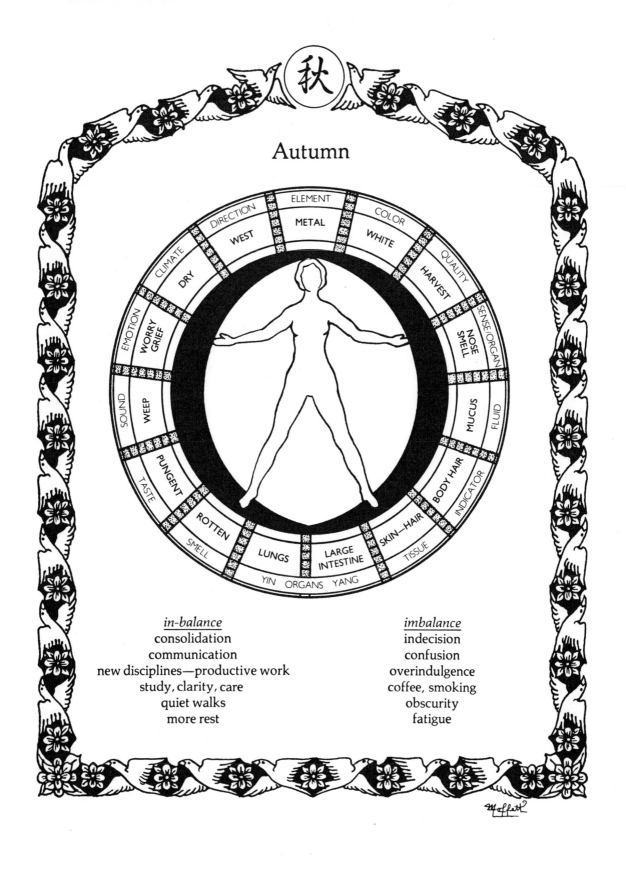

Autumn

ELEMENT METAL
DIRECTION WEST
COLOR WHITE
CLIMATE DRY
QUALITY HARVEST
EMOTION WORRY GRIEF
SENSE ORGAN NOSE SMELL
SOUND WEEP
FLUID MUCUS
TASTE PUNGENT
INDICATOR BODY HAIR
SMELL ROTTEN
TISSUE SKIN–HAIR
ORGANS LUNGS LARGE INTESTINE
YIN ORGANS YANG

in-balance
consolidation
communication
new disciplines—productive work
study, clarity, care
quiet walks
more rest

imbalance
indecision
confusion
overindulgence
coffee, smoking
obscurity
fatigue

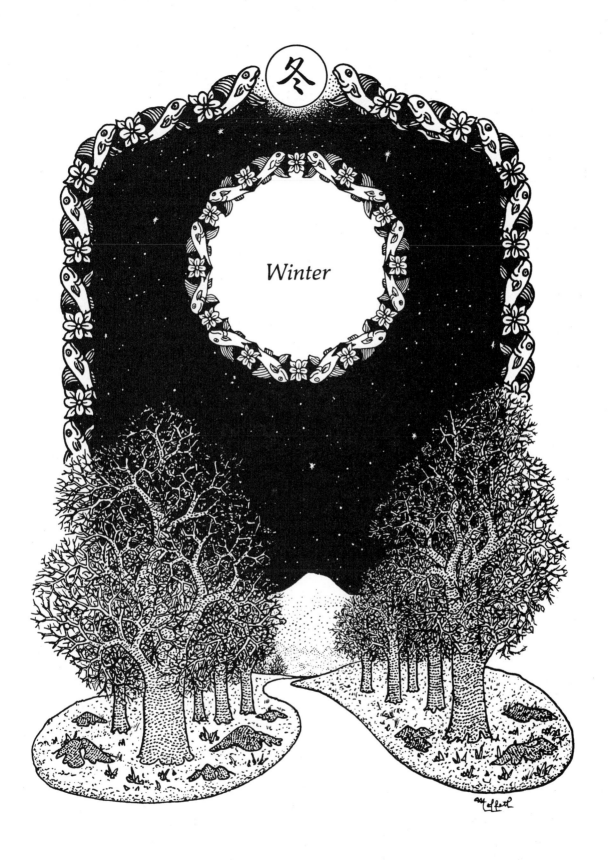

Winter

Feeling Winter

ARE YOU FEELING MORE EMOTIONAL these days? Winters are like that, a more inward and sensitive time. Nature is in her resting season, quiet, withdrawn, deep in the earth and the roots, preparing for spring. You also may be deeper within yourself, seeking replenishment, resting, reflecting, and being more aware of your senses. As the winter climates of cold and wet (snow, rain, or fog) chill you to your bones, seek inner warmth and spend more time at home with family and friends.

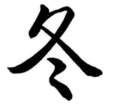

December 21st is the date of the winter solstice, the first day of winter and the day of the longest night. There will be more and more light from now on. Winter seems to be a time to stay active in order to keep your body warm and your energy moving; it is also a time to get plenty of rest, good nutrition, relaxation, and sleep. Dream time is very important to replenishing yourself.

Water Element

According to the Chinese Five Element system, winter is related to the element Water. Are you aware that there has been the same amount of water on the planet since its beginning? Energy can be neither created nor destroyed—only transformed. Water is in the air, on and within the earth, and constitutes a major part of all living matter. This fluid is very adaptable, taking the shape of its container and changing form

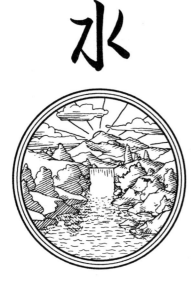

"(In winter) people should re-tire early at night and rise late in the morning and they should wait for the rising of the sun."

NEI CHING

with cold and heat. It supports your being, both as a drink and when carrying you on a boat, a raft, or when swimming.

Water is the essential medium of your body, through which all things pass. This fluid of life is important for functions like the circulation of blood, which carries heat and nourishment throughout the body; the lymphatic flow, which helps to process and eliminate wastes and provides your ability to fight off infections and other foreign agents; and for the flow of urine, saliva, perspiration, tears, and sexual fluids.

Living near the ocean, I watch its ever-changing states and experience its power, its flow, its potential violence, and its peace. Water can be warm and loving, or cold and frightening. It is nourishing, refreshing, and invigorating. By looking at the element, Water, you can see the analogy between the human body and the planet Earth. They both consist of 70–80 percent water. In fact, sea water is almost identical to blood plasma. Water is the circulatory system of the Earth. Clouds, mountain snow, lakes, rivers, streams, and the oceans are all part of this water circulation.

Winter is the season in which the Water element is most dominant. The bladder and kidneys, which deal with the body's water, are the organs associated with the Water element and winter season.

Winter's power is deep and *yin.* It is a time to conserve energy and resources and not be wasteful with your active, outward (*yang*) energy. You need special care in the form of nutrition, warmth, and rest.

The climate associated with the Water element is cold, and its direction is, appropriately, north. The kidneys are nourished by the cold climate, but extreme coldness or wetness can injure them. You must keep yourself warm and dry, especially in the winter, for those cold, wet days can bring out a deep stiffness or pain, especially in the back.

The flavor or taste associated with this element is salty. Most water is actually salty; even in your body, the water contains many mineral salts. If people crave the flavor of salt or really dislike it, they may have a Water imbalance. And eating too much salt creates a craving for water and may injure the kidneys. The *Nei Ching* says that too much salt will "injure the blood," and the blood is correlated with the Fire element and the heart, which directly affects the kidneys. In Western medicine as well, too much salt is seen as the cause of water retention, high blood pressure, and kidney and heart trouble.

The Water element can be related to the emotions in general, but the specific emotional imbalance associated with Water energy is fear. This may be manifest as specific phobias; as a general anxiety about life; or as paranoia or negativity, in which one always expects the worst. Fear can be either a cause or a consequence of a Water imbalance. An illness affecting the bladder or kidneys may generate a fearful feeling; and fear can itself injure these organs, according to the Chinese system. During excitement or in change, one who has a Water imbalance may respond by trembling. This trembling represents a release of fearful energy and tensions. And although fear may block the expression of love, love and faith can transmute fear.

The ears are the sense organ associated with the Water element, so that its sense is hearing. Remember that Water is the receptive element, which listens to sound and is open to energy input. It's interesting that the kidneys and ears are shaped similarly, as is the human embryo. The embryo, and later the fetus, grows in the water medium, through which sounds travel to its developing ears. In traditional Chinese medicine, problems of the ears or hearing may reflect a Water element disharmony.

Two additional associations of the Water element are the groaning sound, and the bones of the body. Groaning, or moaning, comes from deep within, and hearing its overtones in the voice may point to an imbalance in the Water element. Bones and bone marrow are body parts governed by this element. This includes all the bones: the skull, the extremities and the spine, as well as the teeth and the bone marrow (the bone's inner contents where cells are produced and used for growth and renewal in our bodies).

It is said that the kidneys govern the storage of the life force in the bones and marrow. People with bone problems may have a Water imbalance, while a healthy Water element keeps the bones well and strong. Expressions like, "I felt it in my bones," or, "She cries in her bones," suggest the relationship of the bones to deep emotional experiences. The winter is a good time to seek deeper and more intense body therapy to help get to those meaningful and emotional levels.

The Water element also relates to the sex organs and the sexual functions in the body. It rules over the genital and reproductive organs, and the urethral and anal orifices. It also

"The kidneys are the rulers over winter. Kidneys and bladder are related and have to be treated as one in acupuncture. Within the kidneys', 'essence' is stored, and they govern all that is secluded and dormant and that is hoarded up. Their condition is disclosed in the bones and head hair."

CHINESE FOLK MEDICINE

relates to the urine and the sexual secretions. The health of the Water element affects the energy flow during the sexual act, and the health of the function of reproduction. Sexual fluids help lubricate and protect the sperm and egg. Problems like impotence or infertility may arise from a Water imbalance. An excess of sex and resulting congestion, as well as a lack of expression of sexual energy, may affect the kidneys and the balance of the Water element too. Healthy sexual relations require giving and receiving, or *yang* and *yin*, of both partners.

Each of the twelve meridians has the energy flowing through it predominantly two hours each day, as it circulates through the body. Bladder time is from 3 to 5 P.M., and kidney is from 5 to 7 P.M. (see chart for other meridians). This four-hour period of the day is definitely a transition time, getting out of school, or work, and the time when sunset occurs and we prepare for night. During this period of the day we often need a little relaxation to become more receptive. Also it can be a more emotional time for many of us. People who have a difficult time during these hours may reveal a Water imbalance, while those who do well and enjoy this late afternoon/early evening time are probably healthy in this element.

Moon-Water-Emotions

Water must stay in motion; it has a rhythm, a cycle which is primarily ruled by the movement and gravitational pull of the moon. The daily expansions and contractions of the oceans in the tides is like the breathing cycle of the Earth. The moon is *yin*, the receptive, feminine, dark principle, relating to the subconscious—the hidden, the emotions. Water in turn has these same characteristics. The state of Water in your body may reflect the state of your emotions. Like the planet, you can also have droughts and floods, stagnant pools and fresh-flowing streams.

We all have our cycles. Many of us have cycles in which held-in emotions are released, like the winter rains. Then, with the new awareness and expression of these feelings comes a real lightening up of our energy. Water, sometimes held in the body along with the emotions, can cause lethargy and slowness, irritability, and an inability to express ourselves.

From the Chinese viewpoint, individuals with deficient Water energy may find it difficult to slow down, relax or rest, with an inability to reflect clearly. A balanced Water element allows fluidity and flow, an ability to rest and nourish oneself and others, to guide perception and reflection, and have a ready expression of feelings such as love. Qualities of compassion, understanding, and responsiveness to needs and feelings of others are often seen as the maternal and feminine aspect of ourselves, and are also characteristics of the Water element.

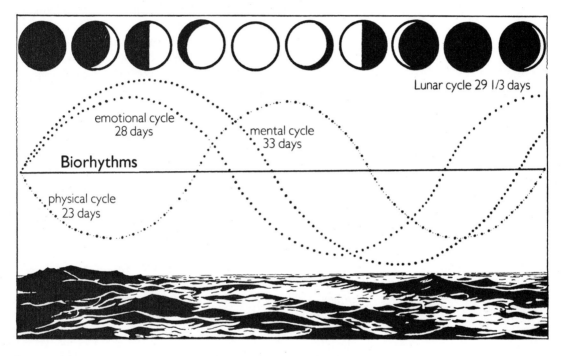

Lunar cycle 29 1/3 days

emotional cycle 28 days

mental cycle 33 days

Biorhythms

physical cycle 23 days

Yin and Yang

The *Oneness* of the universe has two aspects which can be seen as dualities, as polarities, or even as conflicts. These are the two primary forces: *yang*, which seeks to expand into everything, and *yin*, which contracts or seeks nothingness, according to the Chinese system. Both winter and water are the most *yin* parts of their cycles.

Most things exist as a combination of *yin* and *yang*, rather than as purely one or the other. Some aspects of *yin* are: cold, wet, receptive, deep, and inward. *Yin* relates to Earth and to form. *Yang* relates to Heaven and to energy, and is hot, dry, active, light, superficial, and outward.

We see these two forces alternately ebbing and flowing in nature and within our bodies through the year, in the monthly sun-moon cycles, in day and night, and indeed, in each moment—and in our breath and our heartbeats. "Lub-dub," the heart contracts, empties, relaxes, and fills again. The cycles of *yin* and *yang* are like the heartbeat of the universe.

Our awareness follows the same patterns of change. Active awareness, expanding and relating to things outside ourselves, is considered *yang*. Drawing inward, listening, and being receptive, is *yin*. There is a constant shifting balance between the two. Day becomes night, night becomes day, light and darkness. Sunrise and sunset are times of the day when *yin* and *yang* are balanced. Each day, we wake up to the light, slowly unwind from our dream state, expand, and go out for work, activity, and sunshine; meanwhile the *yang* is dominant. Later, we experience *yin* when we come home again for support, nourishment, relaxation, sleep, and the play with inner realities.

Similarly, in each lunar cycle the sun (the male, active, light principle) and the moon (the female, receptive, dark principle) go through many relationships. We experience this cyclical change internally as well. During the time of the new moon (when the sun and moon are in the sky at the same degree relative to earth), with its darker nights, our experience is most *yin*, concerned with inner needs, creativity, and with looking forward into the next cycle. At full moon, when the moon reflects sunlight at night (the sun and moon are 180 degrees apart in the sky relative to earth), our experience is most *yang*, often with bright and active nights, parties, and less need for sleep.

Summer/fall/winter/spring is a *yang/yin* cycle, too—daylight dominates for awhile, then longer nights return. Summer is the most *yang* season, with long days and lots of activity in the sun; then autumn brings increasing *yin*, until the winter solstice. Then, *yang* begins to increase until night and day are even at the spring equinox; and *yang* energy again predominates through the summer. Even though some climates may be warmer or colder, or have less distinct climatic changes, we must realize that the light/dark cycle is the important relationship for differentiating seasons.

During the winter, when the *yin* principle dominates our bodies as well as the climate, this aspect also characterizes the

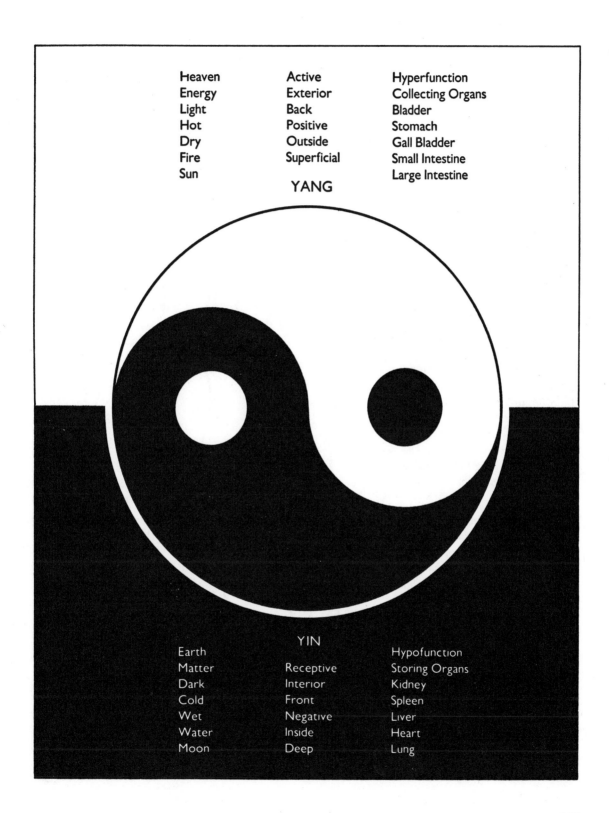

Heaven   Active   Hyperfunction
Energy   Exterior   Collecting Organs
Light   Back   Bladder
Hot   Positive   Stomach
Dry   Outside   Gall Bladder
Fire   Superficial   Small Intestine
Sun   Large Intestine

YANG

YIN

Earth   Hypofunction
Matter   Receptive   Storing Organs
Dark   Interior   Kidney
Cold   Front   Spleen
Wet   Negative   Liver
Water   Inside   Heart
Moon   Deep   Lung

Bladder and Kidney Meridians

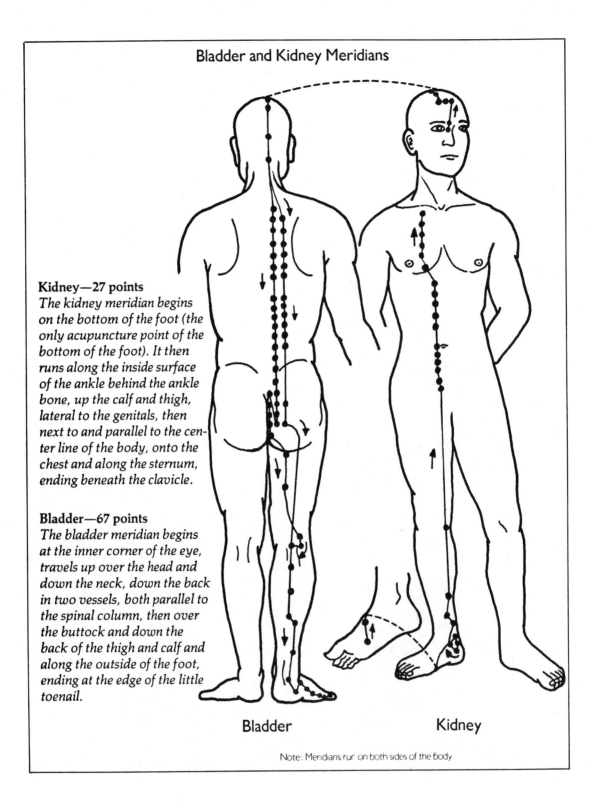

Kidney—27 points

The kidney meridian begins on the bottom of the foot (the only acupuncture point of the bottom of the foot). It then runs along the inside surface of the ankle behind the ankle bone, up the calf and thigh, lateral to the genitals, then next to and parallel to the center line of the body, onto the chest and along the sternum, ending beneath the clavicle.

Bladder—67 points

The bladder meridian begins at the inner corner of the eye, travels up over the head and down the neck, down the back in two vessels, both parallel to the spinal column, then over the buttock and down the back of the thigh and calf and along the outside of the foot, ending at the edge of the little toenail.

Bladder   Kidney

Note: Meridians run on both sides of the body

164

storage function in the body. That is where the deep strength and stamina lie. In fact, the *yin* organs are the deeper, solid organs—liver, heart, lungs, spleen, and kidneys. In contrast, the *yang* principle is hot and dry; in our body, it rules the processing and eliminative aspects, and thus the hollow organs—the large and small intestines, gall bladder, stomach, and bladder.

Bladder and Kidneys

Winter is the strongest *yin* time of the year, and the two organs associated with this season are the kidneys and the bladder, both of which process the most *yin* element, Water.

The bladder is a thick muscular organ in the pelvis which stores and eliminates urine received from the kidneys. The Chinese consider the bladder to be the seat (or storehouse) of the emotions; if it is not functioning well, the rest of the system is stressed.

The bladder's meridian, or energy channel, runs down the back along both sides of the spine. This meridian begins at the inner corners of the eyes, then goes over the head, down the neck and along the spine to the sacrum, and finally travels down the back of the legs to the little toes, where it ends at the 67th point on the outer side of the toenail.

This energy channel is the main one on the back. Tensions and held-in emotions can easily cause congestion in this area and lead to stiffness as well as neck or back pains. So you must keep your back energy loose and flowing through stretching exercises and through freely expressing your feelings.

The kidneys filter the blood and keep the blood and the body clean and in balance. The urine made from filtering the blood passes from the kidneys through the ureters to the bladder and then back to nature via the urethra. The water balance and the acid-base balance in the body are maintained by the kidneys, which extract all kinds of substances from the blood—water; nitrogen compounds like urea and ammonia; minerals and salts, such as sodium, chloride, potassium; and any other chemicals and drugs not needed by the body. Several thousand quarts of blood pass through the kidneys daily, from which 160 quarts of liquid are extracted for further filtering. Most of this liquid is reabsorbed into the body by the

". . . the groins and the bladder are like magistrates of a region or district, they store the overflow and the fluid secretions which serve to regulate vaporization."

NEI CHING

kidney's complex filtering system, leaving one to two quarts to be excreted. The kidneys use this large flow of fluid to collect, concentrate, and eliminate the body's liquid waste.

In the Chinese system, the kidneys are perceived as storing the energy of the life force itself, and are related to birth, life, and death—the cycle of transformation. Look to the kidney energy first if there is chronic illness in the body. As the "seat of the will," willpower itself is seen as coming from the kidneys, which also generate ambition, a desire to do something in one's life. A lack of willpower or ambition may reflect a Water imbalance.

Other organs of elimination besides the kidneys and bladder are the lungs, large intestine, and the skin. The kidneys and the skin both work to clear water from the body. Urine and sweat are both waste products of the blood, and have a similar chemical nature. When the kidneys are clearing toxins poorly or have too much to handle, the skin may have to work harder to help clear these wastes. This can sometimes lead to skin rashes.

High blood pressure is sometimes related to kidney trouble, too. Naboru Muramoto feels strongly that the kidneys may become contracted from the stress of toxic or heavy meat diets. This can lead to poor clearing of the body's water and salts, which in turn increases fluid volume and places more work on the heart. Too much meat or chemical additives may also stiffen or clog up the vascular system, contributing to higher blood pressure and weakening of the heart. In both Chinese and Western medicine, the heart and kidney relationship is a vital one.

To evaluate the health of the kidneys, examine the overall color, clarity, and tone of the skin. A bluish discoloration (or swelling) around the eyes may suggest a Water imbalance and indicate kidney trouble. The color blue is associated with the Water element, relating both to the deep blue sea and to the "blue" feeling of being down emotionally. Being very attracted to blue and wearing it regularly, or else really disliking it, may also signify a Water element imbalance. Instinctively, wearing a certain color a great deal may reveal the body's attempt to strengthen a certain organ or element.

Another diagnostic clue in the Chinese system, relating both to the kidneys and to inner vitality, is the presence of the sparkle of life in the eyes. The vital "life-force" sparkle comes from the kidneys, although the health of the eye tissue itself is related to the liver and Wood element.

The head hair is also a good health indicator for the Water element. Examine the texture and fullness of growth; is it too dry, oily, thick, or thin or balding? Any rapid changes in your hair may suggest an imbalance of the Water element. I believe that premature loss of hair is related to the same high protein, high animal fat diets that affect the kidneys and heart, possibly by clogging hair follicles and leading to poor oxygenation. Your genetic predisposition to specific problems such as balding can be helped or hindered by how you live your life.

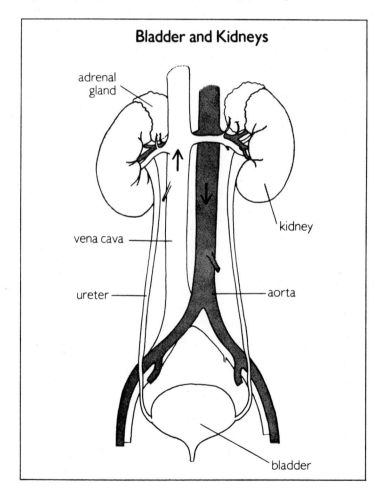

Bladder and Kidneys

adrenal gland

kidney

vena cava

ureter

aorta

bladder

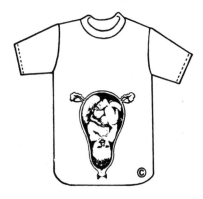

Pregnancy and Birth

Since the kidneys and the Water element are associated with the sexual and reproductive functions, they are related to the process of conception, birth, pregnancy, and mothering. Being receptive, able to listen to others, in touch with feelings, nourishing and loving—are all features important to having a healthy pregnancy and to supporting a child's growth.

The woman's egg must be open to the penetration of a man's sperm. The uterus must be receptive to allowing the fertilized egg to create a home in which to grow—the womb, the container for new life. This growing embryo (and then fetus) survives, supported and protected in a water medium called the amniotic fluid, and is nourished by the mother's blood and thus by her oxygen, nutrition, and vitality. In general, the Chinese consider pregnancy to be a *yin* state for the mother, who must concentrate on her evnironment within, and a *yang* state for the growing, expanding fetus.

The creation of a new human being is an important issue to consider in one's life. Many feel that there is not much greater work or joy than raising a child or children. However, it does require a long-term commitment, the ability to give and to love, and the patience to listen and to teach. Other concerns often interfere with these responsibilities, and many children go through the important early years without the love and support that they need. This love in the early years helps toward inner contentment and the ability to function successfully and lovingly with the outer world.

During pregnancy, the prospective mother usually becomes more *yin*, sensitive, and emotional, all influenced by the increased hormonal output. For a woman to be totally open to entering into this state while pregnant, she needs support from her partner. The man's role during pregnancy traditionally has been supportive, both to provide shelter and food and also to give special care and love to the more sensitive woman. This is still important because excessive *yang* activities for the woman during pregnancy can create pregnancy imbalances and lead to difficulties in a healthy birthing and a healthy baby.

It was necessary for all of us to have had a mother and father in order to arrive here on Earth. Men, women, and children have always needed this magic combination for growth, security, and physical, mental, and emotional health—the loving, nurturing and understanding comfort which has been associated with mothers and the guidance, stability, and care associated with fathers. These are not fixed roles, however; they are continually changing and vary with individuals. Men and women are both able to fill their children's needs.

Traditionally, men often appear more *yang,* or outwardly strong, and women more *yin,* with a deeper emotional strength, which gives them the ability to deal compassionately and effectively with many childhood upsets. But men are becoming more concerned with being aware of and expressing their feelings, providing them with a deeper and more diverse strength and character. This in turn helps to facilitate more meaningful communication between men and women.

There is much to say about pregnancy, birthing, and child-rearing; many relevant and diverse books are presently available on these subjects. A couple of good books if you are interested in learning about yourself, your pregnancy, and especially if you're considering a home birth, are *Spiritual Midwifery* by Ina May Gaskin and the people at The Farm in Tennessee, and *Special Delivery* by Rahima Baldwin. Realize that pregnancy is a state in which a woman needs to give to herself; and a man, to give his partner more support and nurturing. Communication on the emotional level is very important as it can help keep the heart well and the mind at peace.

A truly beneficial and fulfilling experience for two people is to choose to consciously create a child, serving the continuation of humankind. This takes a mutual decision, an understanding of the natural cycle of the woman to know when conception is possible, and clear mental, emotional, physical, and spiritual communication.

Birth Control or Conscious Conception

If one is not prepared to become a parent, there are many ways to prevent getting pregnant. The surest one is to avoid sexual relations with another of the opposite sex. The basic medical approaches for birth control in sexually active people have included birth control pills, the intrauterine device (IUD), the diaphragm and spermicidal jelly, rhythm method, and condoms. All of these have some advantages and some disadvantages, and all are in some way harmful, either by causing specific side effects or by failing to prevent conception. I feel birth control pills are especially dangerous and affect the kidney/Water energy and emotional balance.

Just the concept of birth, or creation, control seems strange. Talk to artists about controlling their expression, and they will tell you about frustration, anger, and pain.

The old "rhythm method," now achieving a more scientific reputation as "natural birth control," is becoming very popular and appears effective if done correctly. It includes the man and woman together taking responsibility, or for a single woman, to understand and follow her fertility cycle, always being aware of when she is in it. This is as useful a tool for getting pregnant as for not, because the woman will learn when she is ovulating. It involves using in combination the "cervical mucus," or Billings "ovulation," method along with observing the basal temperature cycle.

This combined method has been shown in controlled tests in Australia to be 97.7 percent effective. It is described completely in two books, *The Natural Birth Control Book* by Art Rosenblum, and *Natural Birth Control* by Margaret Nofziger.

During a normal menstrual cycle, estrogen stimulates the growth of the uterine wall and, along with follicle-stimulating hormone (FSH), the maturation of an egg, or eggs. For ovulation to occur, the pituitary releases luteinizing hormone (LH) which causes one egg to be released (occasionally two can be released, and if both are fertilized, fraternal twins can result) and raises the body temperature about one degree Fahrenheit.

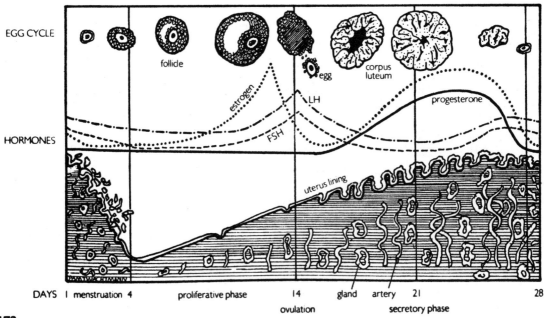

EGG CYCLE

follicle

egg

corpus luteum

estrogen

LH

progesterone

FSH

HORMONES

uterus lining

DAYS   I menstruation 4   proliferative phase   I4   gland   artery   21   28

ovulation   secretory phase

The egg, after leaving the ovary, lives only 12 hours and must have contact with a healthy sperm during that time to be fertilized. This is the only time of the month that a woman is biologically fertile. However, sperm can live from 24–36 hours. So for a woman to be assured of not getting pregnant, she needs to avoid sexual intercourse in the few days before she ovulates, and two days after.

The egg's previous capsule, called the "corpus luteum," makes and secretes *progesterone* after ovulation. This stimulates growth of the uterine wall (the glands and blood vessels) to prepare for the fertilized egg. The secretion of progesterone continues for approximately 14 days. Then if no egg has implanted in the uterine wall, the corpus luteum stops its secretion of progesterone, and the wall and uterine glands break down, resulting in bleeding—the menstrual period.

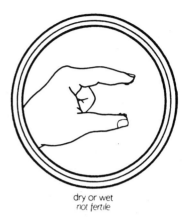

dry or wet
not fertile

The effects of the hormones (estrogen, progesterone, FSH, and LH) create changes which may be learned and followed through the month, so that you can know exactly when your ovulation time will be. This is easier if you have regular menstrual cycles, but even if not, you can know at least the day on which you ovulate.

One thing to do is to follow the body temperature with a basal thermometer. Measure your temperature first thing in the morning upon awakening. It will rise approximately one degree Fahrenheit when ovulation occurs, and will stay at this level until the next menstrual period.

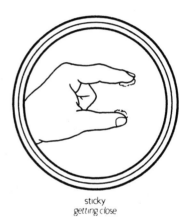

sticky
getting close

Also, the mucus secretions around the cervical opening at the upper portion of the vaginal canal change throughout the month. After the period there is usually only a little mucus, described as "dry." It then changes to being more "wet" and as one gets closer to ovulation the mucus gets "sticky" and then stringy, called "spinn," meaning that if you place some mucus between your thumb and index finger, then pull your fingers apart, the mucus forms threads or strings between them. When stringiness or "spinn" occurs, you are considered fertile and you should not have sexual intercourse that day or for the next two days.

After working with this process for a few months, you can know exactly what your cycle is. When you know your ovulation time, you need to abstain from intercourse at least three days before it and two days after it. Now, this is the catch, because you must know when you are fertile several days

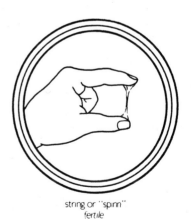

string or "spinn"
fertile

before ovulation. Thus, learning your pattern and abstaining at the appropriate times *should* prevent pregnancy.

Of course, vaginal infections or having sex before checking your mucus may affect the quality of the mucus. Other symptoms that occur with ovulation besides sticky to stringy mucus and the rise in temperature may include breast soreness, "mittelschmerz" (pain secondary to ovulation), increased energy and sexual desire, and oiliness of the hair and skin.

Some proponents of this method of natural birth control also suggest being aware of your "cosmic fertility" time which is based on astrology, specifically the angle that the sun and moon made at the time of your birth. This same angle occurs each month and is also a potentially fertile time which may be different from your physiologic fertile time. There is need for more research on these currently popular methods as well as more education.

If you have irregular cycles and wish to make them more regular, try the process called *Lunaception,* described in the book by Louise Lacey. To describe simply this approach—if you sleep by an indirectly shining low-watt light bulb for several days in the midst of your menstrual cycle, this can help to regulate it. The light simulates the effects of the full moon. This method has even been used to adjust the period and ovulation times to adapt to a certain lunar phase.

Read one of the natural birth control books on the ovulation, mucus, and temperature methods before trying to put them into practice. It is very important that you know what you are doing.

Abortion

If you don't know what you are doing and misuse your method of birth control or use none at all while having sexual intercourse, you may find yourself in a difficult situation. There is the potential, besides the joys of pregnancy and birth, for great frustration, sadness, anger, and spiritual upset when a woman and man find themselves having to choose a "therapeutic abortion."

Sadly, the responsibility to deal with this problem has often fallen on the shoulders of the woman. Each of us must choose for ourselves what we will do with our lives at any given moment, but the abortion of pregnancy should not be taken lightly. It may have physical, mental, and many emotional and spiritual side effects. It is never painless, yet oftentimes it is the best way out of a difficult situation.

Any concerned woman or man unable to bear the responsibility of full parenthood will not wish to bring a child into an unbalanced home environment. So pregnancy can also be an unconscious creation which must be stopped midway.

Why do people have unwanted pregnancies and abortions? It has to do with sexual activity of course, but, like an illness, it also gives us a chance to take a look and understand ourselves better. In a sense, an unconscious desire is seeking to be known and become conscious.

Some women become pregnant easily while others often take months or years to conceive. This obviously involves both individual makeup, also appropriate preparation and the development of deep receptivity on the part of the woman, which depends on her sense of commitment and openness felt toward her partner. A pregnancy can create or strengthen bonds between the people involved.

Many women have told me they felt their primary form of conception control was mental. The mind can create barriers and is often harder to penetrate than the sensitive heart. If a woman binds herself in her mind to a man, and this may even be subconsciously, she may be more liable to become pregnant. If she doesn't feel this emotional and spiritual bond deeply, it may be more difficult to conceive. Mind you, this is a purely intuitive hypothesis, but it is an interesting one to look at. The positive aspect of bonding such as sensing another's feelings and being receptive to them may be associated with the energy of the Water element, and thus influence the ability for healthy reproduction.

On a spiritual level, abortions can cause confusion, and what I believe are karmic actions, meaning they cause certain reactions which may appear as difficulties. Karma is a process of learning from this natural law of the universe. Each life crisis or illness has a lesson which, if we learn, we will not need to experience again. Yet, if we deny the potential learning this experience represents, the same lesson will present itself again and again, often more intensely, until we learn it. I have seen some women who have had a therapeutic abortion at one time, only to have difficulties or a spontaneous abortion or miscarriage in their next "wanted" pregnancy. Communication clears karma and learning our lessons will help prevent difficulties. Becoming responsible for our sexuality and its outcomes is a beginning.

When a woman becomes pregnant, she is filled with a spirit of a new being. If she alters the physical process, it is still important to receive the message that this being is bringing to the world. Communication with the spirit of the baby is possible and has been described by many women (see *Hygieia-A Woman's Herbal* by Jeannine Parvati). In an abortion, the woman or the prospective parents are choosing to grow and give birth to themselves instead of to another being, but in this instance they must incorporate an awareness of the being that came briefly to inhabit their lives.

Another hypothesis is that although a woman may have a physical end of pregnancy she and her body continue to be pregnant on other levels. She will, of course, need to replenish herself physically, but also she may be more emotionally sensitive and more in need of support in the months following abortion. Many times, these women have a difficult time emotionally or physically during the period around the time they would have delivered. I saw two women in my practice who incurred physical injury around their due dates. One even fell from her horse and fractured her pelvis. She called me right after it happened. I told her to go to the hospital for x-rays, and then the sparks went off in my brain and I remembered that she had had an abortion with much conflict months before. I asked her when her due date from that conception was. She thought and answered, "today." This incident brought to me the awareness that I have just stated. This is not meant to be a scare tactic or to suggest that it happens a lot, but it should be something that is considered under those circumstances. I would like to see studied the relationship between women's health around their estimated time of delivery after abortion.

I now tell a woman who has just had an abortion to care for herself as if she were still pregnant. She needs to eat well, rest, get proper exercise and fresh air, and give herself special nurturing. She should continue to be aware of the process of pregnancy and her emotional sensitivity, and take the week around her would-be delivery time to be with herself, or her partner if that is relevant, and to be open to any changes or new awareness she may experience.

Winter Diet

As you move into winter, you need to adjust your diet once again. The weather is colder, so a diet that produces more heat is necessary. Days are shorter and you tend to have less physical activity, thereby burning fewer calories than you might during the more active summer. Don't increase your food intake too much or you may gain more weight than you wish. A diet which is mainly carbohydrate and protein will produce the heat you need and perhaps give you a few added pounds, but with even moderate activity, you should stay in pretty good shape until spring comes and you can once again cleanse and lighten up.

Fruits are less available and form only a small part of the winter diet unless you live in a tropical climate. Vegetables can be eaten daily, some as salad, and others in cooked form, either steamed or baked. Some fried or sauteed foods fit more with the winter diet than in other seasons, though too much heated oil is hard on the liver. An occasional vegetable casserole might be good, too. Vegetable soups, especially on a cold or wet day, are nutritious, warming, and easy to digest. Since nature's plants are in their deeper parts, root vegetables like carrots, turnips, onions, and potatoes are especially right for the winter diet. Garlic and ginger root will spice up your life, too, and cayenne pepper adds heat to your meals and warmth to your toes!

Cooked whole grains make an excellent staple in the winter diet. These complex carbohydrates burn well in the body as fuel and are good for the intestines and for elimination. Millet and buckwheat are good body heaters and less starchy than the other grains like brown rice, wheat, barley, or oats. If grains are cooked or eaten with beans like red aduki beans, mung beans, black beans, or lentils, you will have a complete protein. Muramoto states that red aduki beans are good for the kidneys while black beans assist the sexual functions.

Millet and black beans (soak beans in water for 12 hours before cooking with millet) or brown rice, lentils, and sunflower seeds (ratio 2:1:1) can be cooked together by simmering slowly in one and a half times their amount of water. After about 40 minutes, dish out the mixture into bowls, and add a little fresh oil, tamari, cayenne, and nutritional yeast, or yogurt, curry, and parsley, and eat up. These grains and bean mixtures make complete vegetable proteins and are tasty, warming, and nutritious. Complete proteins contain all the essential amino acids which your body does not produce.

Nuts are good in the winter as a snack or in salads. You can make nut milks too, as described in the Late Summer section. Cow or goat milk products can be eaten somewhat more freely than in other seasons. Feta cheese, which is made from sheep's milk, is one of the easier ones for your body to handle. It breaks apart rather than sticks together and the slightly salty flavor fits in with the winter diet.

For meat eaters, I would recommend primarily fish, particularly deep-sea fish like halibut and swordfish from nonpolluted areas. Some chicken or red meat might be okay if you are sure the animals have not been fed with lots of chemicals and hormones to pump up their muscles. Occasional red meat stimulates and brightens up the blood, heart, and complexion, and is a great building food, but too much is over-stimulating and endangers the heart, blood vessels, and kidneys. After you begin eating less meat in your diet, you'll become more aware of what effect it has on you.

The winter climate varies from place to place, with different degrees of coldness, wetness, and sunshine. You each have your own level of activity which varies as well. On a day-to-day basis the climate and your activities may change, but your body will tell you what to consume. You must listen.

Ocean Food

Since winter is related to the Water element, let us look into the deep blue sea to find more healthful foods. I just mentioned ocean (salt water) fish, low in fats with high amounts of protein, minerals and vitamins, as a very good food source. Another great source of nutrition is ocean seaweed. Seaweeds are very common in the Japanese diet.

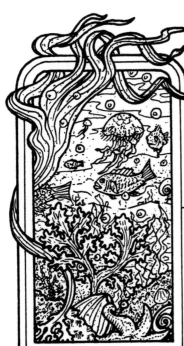

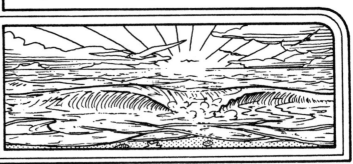

Seaweeds like kelp, dulse, nori, and hijiki are high-protein vegetables, high in vitamins E and A, and particularly rich in calcium, phosphorus, potassium, iron, iodine and other trace minerals. They stimulate and strengthen the skin, hair and nails, and nourish the endocrine system, especially the thyroid and adrenal glands. Seaweeds can be eaten raw after rinsing off the salt, but they may be very chewy that way. Most often, they are eaten in soups, toasted to eat with rice or vegetables, or wrapped around rice with vegetables or fish, as in sushi. Sushi is a Japanese dish in which nori seaweed is wrapped around white rice with the center containing a piece of raw fish, cucumber, or white radish.

There is even a seaweed product put out as a powder, sodium alginate, which when taken orally in capsules or tablets, two/twice daily, is supposed to assist the body in eliminating accumulated radiation and other heavy metals and toxins.

There is a wholesome sushi dish which was invented by Bethany ArgIsle, called "deep-sea divers." Boil up a medium sized pot of brown rice. Into a wooden bowl, place several chopped yellow or white onions and 4–6 pressed cloves of garlic; cover the onions and garlic with cold-pressed olive oil, then squeeze two small or medium-sized lemons, add a taste of honey or pure maple syrup, some cayenne pepper or hot sauce without preservatives, then add soy sauce, tamari, or miso to taste, and a splash of spring water or sake. Into this bowl add the brown rice and mix.

Now you'll need about two packages of nori seaweed sheets to roll around that flavorful rice. Lay out one sheet of nori and place a couple of tablespoons of rice across the center. Along the top of the rice you can run cilantro (sprouted coriander), shredded or slivered daikon (white radish), or alfalfa sprouts. "Kim chee," Korean spiced cabbage, can also be used in the center if you like your sushi hot. Then roll it up.

Each "diver" should be about 1-1/2 inches in diameter. Lay your "deep-sea divers" on a tray, cover, and refrigerate. After 8–12 hours, they will have congealed, the seaweed will be tender, and you can cut them into 2–4 inch lengths and serve. This sweet and sour version should be a big hit!

Soybeans, Tofu, and Miso

The soybean is another food whose use is growing rapidly. It is an inexpensive, high-protein (35–40 percent) food which is particularly important to the vegetarian since it is one of the few sources of complete protein and a good substitute for animal foods. It is still best, though, to obtain your protein from a variety of sources.

Soybeans can be sprouted, cooked as the whole bean, or used to make soymilk, tofu, and miso. They are not only rich in protein, but also high in many minerals like calcium, phosphorus, and potassium, with moderate amounts of iron, B vitamins and other trace elements.

Tofu is soybean curd, and for a simple home recipe soak the whole beans 36–48 hours, changing the water every 12 hours. Then rinse and blend the beans with a little water and pour into a pot of boiling water. Bring beans to boil and let cool. Then add nigari or lemon juice to coagulate. Let it sit for about 12 hours and the curd and whey will separate and both can be used, but the curd (tofu) made into cakes is more popular. Tofu is a tasty, nutritious protein food, with a cheese-like quality, but is much lighter than cheese. It goes well with most any vegetable dish and with grains, especially brown rice. Steamed, baked, or lightly fried in oil or water with other vegetables, it can be used in many ways. Onions, carrots, celery, tofu, and cashew nuts or sliced almonds all cooked together make a tasty dish. Tofu is great added to salads, or makes a wonderful salad dressing when blended with oil, lemon, avocado, a bit of miso, and seasonings.

A tofu-avocado salad is a refreshing, filling, high-protein treat. Mash a half pound of uncooked tofu with one or two avocados, add a little ground sunflower seed/nut mix, a little olive oil, diced green onion and tomato, fresh lemon, seasonings like soy sauce, cayenne pepper, yeast, and basil. This can be eaten as it is, in a whole grain bread sandwich with alfalfa sprouts, or as a dip for chips, crackers, celery or carrot sticks.

Miso is another important soybean product, also known as soybean paste. The soybeans are fermented and aged alone or with grains such as brown rice or barley to make several kinds of miso. It is an important part of the Japanese diet as a soup base, and its use is growing rapidly in America. It is rich in protein and vitamins and contains about ten percent salt.

Miso is an alkalinizing food and its fermentation assists the body's digestion and metabolism. In Japan it is also said to improve one's resistance to illness. For those who wish to strengthen their systems, miso can be used daily as a broth, as it is said to be a good tonic. A teaspoon to a cup of boiling water is mixed. Do not boil miso as it can get very bitter and this destroys the living bacteria and enzymes. In Oriental medicine, miso has been used in the treatment of arthritis, colitis, diabetes, and hypoglycemia; for tobacco problems; and to assist in breast feeding. It is a great afternoon drink for those who suffer from late afternoon or post-work symptoms like headache, dizziness, irritability, or general low energy.

A good soup to have on the fire for your friends and family on a rainy day will combine the winter foods in a miso broth. Simmer some carrots, onions and garlic in water in a stainless steel, porcelain, earthenware or iron pot for 15–20 minutes. then turn off the fire, add miso paste, a good squeeze of lemon, and whatever seasonings you wish. Stir, cover, and let the pot sit and cool for 30 minutes or so until it reaches a warm edible temperature. I like to add pieces of mochi, which is made from sweet glutinous rice and mugwort herb. It really thickens the soup and adds yet another nice flavor.

With the comtemporary concern over x-rays and other forms of environmental radiation, you should know that both miso and seaweed are said to act in the body to help rid it of radiation, heavy metals like lead and strontium, and other toxic substances. In Hiroshima after the bombings, one hospital which served miso every day to all its patients observed a much lower incidence of radiation sickness and death than in the general population or at other hospitals.

Salt

All these highly mineralized ocean products come from the salty sea, and are good sources for our daily salt needs. Sodium chloride, NaCl, is considered the basic body salt, though any combination of a positively charged element(s) with a negatively charged one(s) makes a salt, such as calcium phosphate $Ca_3(PO_4)_2$, the bone salt, or potassium chloride, KCl. Sodium chloride is one of our key body salts and aids in the distribution of water throughout the body. It is called the "electric salt" as it helps to circulate the current of life.

As vital as it is to human life, salt (NaCl) can also be a danger, especially in the amounts eaten in the average diet. Western medicine has observed its involvement in diseases like hypertension and congestive heart failure. Excess salt, creating water retention, can cause emotional problems and affect the kidneys' work in balancing body water. Salt use is commonly related to premenstrual tensions. Too much in the diet can create constipation as well.

"The minerals and enzymes contained in seaweeds aid the body in eliminating the effects of animal food and help it adapt to vegetal-quality foods. In addition, seaweed helps the body discharge radioactive wastes imbibed from the atmosphere (food environment too)! It has been proven experimentally that alginic acid, an important element in brown algae such as wakame, kombu, other types of kelp, and hijiki, acts on metallic elements in the intestines, turning them into insoluble salts which are discharged from the body."

HEALING OURSELVES
Naboru Muramoto

179

It is actually the sodium of the sodium chloride that creates the main effect. Sodium is the key element in the blood and the fluids surrounding the cells, and takes water with it wherever it goes. Other sodium chemicals like monosodium glutamate, used commonly in Chinese cooking and responsible for many postmeal symptoms, and sodium nitrite, a carcinogen used to preserve cured meats, can create similar imbalances.

In Oriental medicine, it is thought that the right amounts of naturally occurring salts give power, strength, and energy, and support the kidneys and the Water element. However, too much weakens us and overworks the kidneys. A diet high in red meats and animal fats carries much concentrated salt and oil which over a long period affects the fine blood filtering membranes of the kidneys and thus, their function. Both this diet and too much salt also can injure the blood, leading to vessel and heart problems. It is possible that salt, NaCl, is only of secondary concern to these other dietary dangers.

The body sometimes stores excessive amounts of salt. Some ways to eliminate this is to diminish the consumption of animal meats for a while in the diet and consume more fruits and raw vegetables. Also, a little alcohol helps clear salt which is possibly why meat eaters crave alcohol so often. Bathing, especially in a mineral bath or the ocean, helps to eliminate stored salt from the body.

Our bodies need approximately 500–1,000 milligrams of salt per day. This is less than a teaspoonful, but naturally occurring salts found in foods, both animal and vegetable, when spread through the day, can be handled more easily.

Nowadays, processing foods removes much of their natural salts, and then, for flavor, manufacturers add more salt (white sugar too) to many of these foods. Almost all packaged and canned foods have some salt added to them. This chemical can create physical and psychological addiction just as sugar does, and it starts early, as many commercial baby foods have added salt. Even the water of most cities has significant levels of sodium. Some cities in Texas, Missouri, California, Arizona, and New Mexico have very high levels of sodium in the public drinking water.

The table salt that most people consume is not good because it is refined through heat processing, bleached with chemicals to make it white, then another chemical, aluminum stearate, is added so that the salt flows well and doesn't clump. Natural salts like sea or rock salt crystals will stick together when they become moist. Sea water is about three percent NaCl and you can buy good sea salt in which sunshine alone has been used to extract it. I think this is the best salt to use if you have to use salt, but you must use it sparingly as it is concentrated.

There are some good vegetable salts made of dried and powdered vegetables with some sea salt added; some are even made with low sodium concentrations. A high-protein form of salt flavoring is made from sesame seeds and sea salt. It is called sesame salt, or gomasio, and is made by toasting sesame seeds lightly and quickly in a dry skillet, then grinding them in a coffee or nut grinder, and mixing with sea salt. Use seven or more parts sesame to one part sea salt. Sesame seeds are a high calcium/mineral food and a good one for people who eat little animal products.

Most soy sauce sold in stores is mass-produced and contains preservatives. However, "tamari" soy sauce is a naturally aged and fermented preparation from soybeans, with only wheat, salt and water. It is flavorful, about 18 percent salt, and can be used sparingly. It is especially tasty for grain dishes. Miso paste made in the USA is about ten percent salt, but when used in soups it dilutes to about one percent, even though it has a salt-quenching taste. You do need some daily salt in your diet, and the more you exercise and sweat, the more replacement of salt you need. Miso broth and soup are good ways to do this.

In general, however, it is best to try to get most of your salt intake from the wide selection of nature's foods in which sodium chloride and other salts occur. It is not easy to break the habit of adding salt to your foods. It is very important to stop using refined table salt and products made with added salt. The fewer spices and added salts and sugars you use in your diet, the more sensitive your palate will become to the inherent taste of foods, and the more you and your body will enjoy these foods and the benefits that come with them.

Exercise

Winter is the season of storage and preparation. You need to take special care with your activity level during the winter months. This is a busy time, with the holidays and all, but you

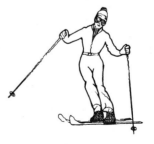

must be careful not to run your batteries down. Plenty of sleep and relaxation from tensions will help to recharge you. Though this is a time of less physical activity, you still must keep your body in shape. *Move every joint every day!* Exercise, stretching, and dance forms which require good, deep breathing will help keep your energy circulating.

Deep breathing actually requires the use of your abdominal muscles to fully expand the lungs, filling their lower and upper parts. A complete exhalation empties the lungs via contracting the abdominal muscles. Complete breathing fully exercises the diaphragm, your breathing muscle. Air is most important to life; you can live a long time without food, days without water, but only a few minutes without air. "Life is in the breath, therefore he who only half breathes, half lives," a Yoga proverb tells us.

The more you can get your energy circulating, open up your joints, and release your resistances, the more your body will clear out its excesses, such as too much food, drugs, emotions, work, tensions, etc. You will then feel lighter and better, stronger and clearer, and have more command of your creative, expressive, and communicative being. Two processes which will help you produce these results are ancient Eastern practices: *Yoga* from India, and *tai chi chuan* from China.

Yoga

Yoga is a multi-leveled discipline that generates health and flexibility. It can range from being simply a series of daily exercises called "asanas," or postures, to a total life style incorporating the regular practice of physical exercises or "asanas," meditation, diet and life philosophy. Yoga is a Sanskrit word meaning "union" or "joining together," as in integrating the body, mind, and spirit. Its root is "to yoke" as to control or guide the mind. B.K.S. Iyenger, author of *Light on Yoga*, gives an analogy between the mind and a chariot, both being pulled by two forces, the animal and the breath. This analogy also applies to the Chinese system, relating the lungs (breath), the mind, and the animal spirit which represents the instincts and desires. By controlling the breath, we gain the strength to tame the desires and bring peace to the mind. A way to do this is by disciplined and regular practice of yoga called "sadhana."

Creating new habits will help to replace the older ones. By practicing asanas (yoga postures) regularly, you can develop

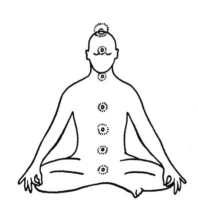

balance and agility, endurance, strength, and wonderful vitality. Yoga helps to relieve stress, bring relaxation, and maintain emotional harmony. It also helps to relieve stiffness in the joints, limbs, and spine. This is important to how you feel: a yoga proverb says "you are as young as your spine is flexible."

Many people tell me that doing yoga helps them center themselves and puts them in touch with their bodies. Focusing the mind on the movements, as in deep concentration, helps you to feel the whole body and its areas of tension, and to relax and release these tensions. Yoga is wonderful for arthritis and as physical therapy for many illnesses. In stimulating the life force (prana) you increase your body's healing powers, vitality, and strength.

There are many, many yoga postures, styles, and teachers. It is not a competitive sport. You must go at your own pace and watch and listen to your body. Each stretch is only that, a stretch, not a painful push. Joel Kramer, yoga teacher, calls yoga practice "playing the edge," finding how far you can go, the edge of your abilities. It creates subtle changes that you will notice. Use a flat floor or earth surface covered with a rug, a foam mat, or a folded blanket. Allow minimally 20–30 minutes daily for the exercises and relaxation. Wear comfortable, loose clothing. The early morning is a common time to practice, though you may find that your body is stiffer earlier in the day. Late afternoon or evening is also a good time, or even before bedtime, but you should practice on an empty stomach, at least two hours after a meal.

During pregnancy, most postures can be done the first few months; then more care must be observed. Two books that describe some good yoga postures for pregnancy are *Prenatal Yoga* by Jeannine Medvin and *Spiritual Midwifery* by Ina May Gaskin. During menstrual periods in women, certain inverted postures are sometimes not recommended.

There are many books of yoga with pictures to display the many techniques and positions. In every city there are practitioners and teachers of yoga. It is best to have first-hand experience in learning a "set" which you can continue. This can be done in a couple of months. Discipline and continuation is up to you. Some books which are good teachers include Richard Hittleman's *Yoga: 28 Day Exercise Plan* and Swami Kriyananda's *Yoga Postures for Self-Awareness*. Both are simple, straightforward, and good for beginners. A more advanced but inclusive book is *Light on Yoga*, by B.K.S. Iyengar, who

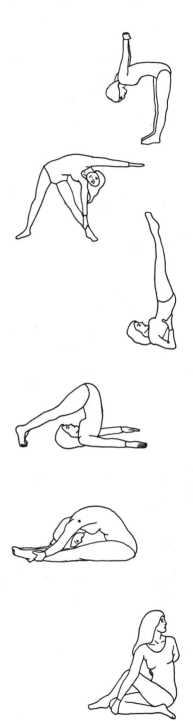

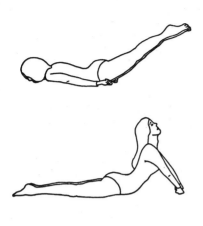

demonstrates his own amazing flexibility. There are a few good yoga books designed for the elderly, one being *Easy Does It: Yoga for People Over 60* by Christensen and Rankin. A yoga book for children that is also fun is *Be a Frog, Be a Bird, Be a Tree*, by Rachel Carr.

You don't have to see the old image of yoga as being done by foreigners who go through many strange contortions or advanced postures like headstands or "full lotus" position. There is a place to start for each of you, but remember, go at your own pace. Yoga includes many gentle exercises geared toward complete breathing, relaxation, and gentle stretching.

These might include sitting cross-legged and breathing; lying flat on your back for deep relaxation, "savasana;" forward, backward, and side-to-side bending. As you gain comfort and flexibility, you can advance into such positions as the cobra, locust, leg clasp, plough, and shoulder stand. Most poses have beginning and intermediate stretches. The inverted poses like the head or shoulder stand, and the plough, and the abdominal lifts (sucking in the abdomen) all help to stimulate the abdominal organs, and especially the glands like the thyroid, allowing yoga to help reduce and regulate body weight.

Winning has to do with nothing other than feeling good about yourself.

Yoga generally enhances circulation and the functions of the organs, glands, and nervous system. And yoga is truly geared toward realizing the Self as it reawakens the great power that lies dormant in the organism and utilizes it for developing one's potential.

Tai Chi Chuan

Tai chi chuan, a flowing series of movements, is an ancient Oriental art used for self-defense, flexibility, and health. It means "the supreme ultimate" and is symbolized by the *yin-yang* symbol, for it promotes centering and harmony—a blending of the inner and outer, the mind and body, masculine and feminine. With these effects, tai chi is often considered a form of meditation and a martial art. It creates power and strength as well as grace and flexibility. There are a variety of forms and many teachers of this "dance of quiet motion." Books are available with pictures of all the movements, but one must really learn tai chi from an experienced teacher.

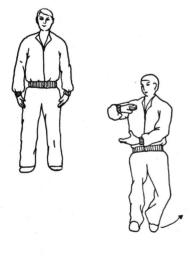

The effects toward balance and coordination are subtle, but powerful. There are short forms with 64 movements and longer ones with 108 movements. Tai chi can be done slowly or quickly. Its origin is linked to the *I Ching, the Book of Changes,* an ancient Chinese text describing 64 different social situations and the possible changes that exist in nature. Tai chi chuan has names for its moves like "waving hands like clouds," "single whip," "grasping sparrows tail," and "repulsing the monkey." It is beautiful to watch, and replenishing to do.

It brings a sense of flowing like a river, a rhythm that simulates that of nature, and a circulation of the "chi," or life force energy (called "prana" in India). From the back cover of *Tai Chi—A Way of Centering and I Ching* by Gia-Fu Feng and Jerome Kirk,

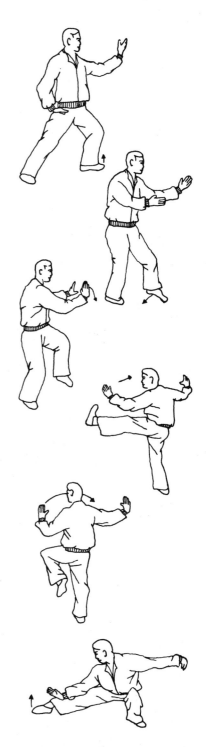

"(Tai chi is) Meditation in movement, a philosophical system, a set of principles of self-defense, a prophylaxis against disease, and exquisite dance. It corrects your posture and enhances relaxation. It energizes your body and tranquilizes your spirit. It is a bridge between Eastern meditation and Western psychotherapy, integrating mind and senses. The effortless effort of its movements leads to the action of non-action and the ancient message of the I Ching."

Tai chi chuan and yoga are more subtle forms of exercise than many Western sports. In winter, inner strengthening is important, especially helpful in clearing the possible body stagnation. As the seasons change, your activities and exercises will also change, but the balance of the inward-directed, stretching and the outward-oriented activities must always be present. Remember, the *yin* and *yang* energies exist together as one; to be dominantly one or the other allows you to experience only part of life.

Each one of you has your own exercise rhythm. To learn a new practice, you might begin with the traditional form taught by an experienced teacher, then allow your own expression to happen. Both yoga and tai chi are body languages which mirror the movements of nature. They began somewhere, very likely with someone like you or me sitting around, who became inspired. The creative potential of the human being is beautiful and never-ending. If you observe children playing, you can see their flexibility and the many yoga-like postures they assume with their only teacher being their spirit of youth.

Herbs

During the winter, when much of the energy is in the roots of plants, boiling up some herbal roots can be helpful for your roots, too. Many herb roots are body and blood cleansers as well, strengthening specific systems. For example, burdock root is good for the blood, lungs, and skin. Comfrey root helps the lungs and mucous linings, especially having a tonic effect on the intestinal walls, increasing your potential for assimilation of nutrients, a most important process for your well-being. You are not necessarily what you eat; more precisely, you are what you assimilate.

During this season marshmallow root (*Althaea officinalis*) is particularly helpful for soothing irritations or inflammation in the kidneys and bladder. This root, made into a tea, and taken internally, acts as a diuretic, increasing the flow of urine, and as a demulcent-emollient, meaning it soothes and softens body tissue. It can be used medicinally as a poultice to heal and allay sore and inflamed areas. A poultice is made by crushing the leaf or root, pouring just enough boiling water over it to make a thick paste and applying it to the appropriate area(s), then covering the poultice and area with a hot cloth or a hot water bottle.

Marshmallow root can be used as well both internally and externally for inflammation of the mucous membranes, especially bladder, vaginal areas, and rectum, or for inflamed bowels. It is also helpful for lung and bronchial complaints.

In winter, you also may need herbs which are body heaters. Cayenne pepper, for example, is a good natural stimulant in winter just as in summer. Ginger root (*Zingiber officinale*) is another good heater as it helps circulation and increases the strength of the Fire element.

Ginger root is simmered 15–20 minutes for tea or used in cooking. It is a stimulating tonic for the stomach, increasing gastric secretions and aiding digestion. It helps to relieve intestinal gases, so it is helpful for digestive cramps and abdominal pains, as well as an herb to remedy diarrhea. As a tea and compress ginger root has been used commonly for colds and bronchitis and for suppressed menstruation. A small towel can be soaked in a strong hot ginger tea and applied to the cold or congested area. When drunk hot as a tea, ginger facilitates sweating, so often helpful for fevers and colds.

Other bladder and kidney herbs include a berry, a seed, and a leaf: juniper berries, flax seeds, and nettle leaves. Juniper (*Juniperus communis*) acts as a carminative (relieves intestinal gas) and a diuretic as well as being helpful in vaginal and venereal diseases. It is good in combination with other diuretic herbs such as cleavers and uva ursi. Juniper berries are used as a preventive against disease when taken after exposure to illness or when resistance is low. The berries chewed or taken as tea can also be used daily when travelling to keep your resistance high.

Flaxseed (*Linum usitatissimum*), simmered and drunk as a tea, is useful in mucous and inflamed conditions and in problems of the urinary organs, soothing and cleansing the kidneys and bladder. Ground flaxseed mixed with water makes a good poultice on local inflammations and boils.

Nettle (*Urtica dioica*) leaves are eaten, drunk as tea, or made into hair shampoo or lotion for the complexion. It is a diuretic, tonic, and astringent and is considered an excellent herb for kidney trouble, backaches, or uterine problems. You can use it as a kidney tonic, building strength and energy when you drink it daily as a tea. Make the tea by adding one cup of boiling water to a pot which has one tablespoon of nettle leaves in it. Steep 20 minutes and drink.

The young leaves lightly steamed and eaten are high in iron, act as a blood purifier, and may assist in weight reduction. The (stinging) nettle plant causes a mild red, itchy skin reaction when used externally, and this action has been helpful for the joint pains of rheumatism.

A few herbal combinations for kidney and bladder problems can use any of these herbs just mentioned. For bladder infections, drink lots of tea made with marshmallow root, juniper berry, cleavers, and peppermint. A nice tea combination for winter is ginger root, flax or fenugreek seeds, and nettle. Fenugreek seed tea is also a good kidney and adrenal tonic and can be brewed with marshmallow root, juniper berries, cleavers, and nettle.

To make super herbal teas, give each herb its proper place in the whole. Leaves and flowers go last in the pot, never boiled, while barks and roots need simmering for 15–20 minutes and seeds for 5–10 minutes to extract their deeper essence before adding and steeping with other leaf and flower herbs in the teapot. Before drinking, let all herbs steep together in a teapot for 20 minutes.

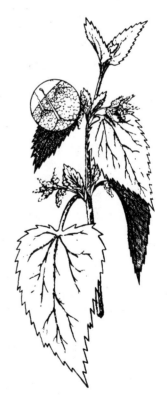

Nettle
Urtica dioica

187

Herbal Tea Preparation

Each herb can best give its essence to the mixture as follows:

Hard roots (e.g. comfrey, burdock)—Simmer 20–30 minutes.

Soft roots (e.g. licorice, marshmallow, ginger)—Simmer 10–15 minutes.

Barks (e.g. cinnamon, sassafras)—Simmer 10–20 minutes.

Seeds or berries (e.g. fennel, fenugreek, anise, juniper)—Simmer 5–10 minutes.

Leaves (e.g. peppermint, rosemary, nettle)—Never boil or simmer! Just place in pot and pour in boiling water. Steep 20 minutes.

Flowers (e.g. hibiscus, chamomile)—Don't cook; steep 10–20 minutes.

Sample Tea

using comfrey root, ginger root, cinnamon bark, fennel seed, peppermint, and chamomile.

To make 4 cups of tea, begin by simmering one full tablespoon of comfrey root in 5 cups of water in a covered stainless steel or glass pot. After 5–10 minutes, add 5 thin slices of ginger root and a few sticks of cinnamon bark. In another 5–10 minutes add a tablespoon of fennel seeds and let herbs simmer together for 5–10 minutes. This makes 20–30 minutes of simmering so far. Now pour all this into a teapot which has in it two tablespoons of peppermint and one tablespoon of chamomile, then let this whole formula steep together for 15–20 minutes. Pour and serve as is, or with a taste of honey and/or a twist of lemon. Enjoy!

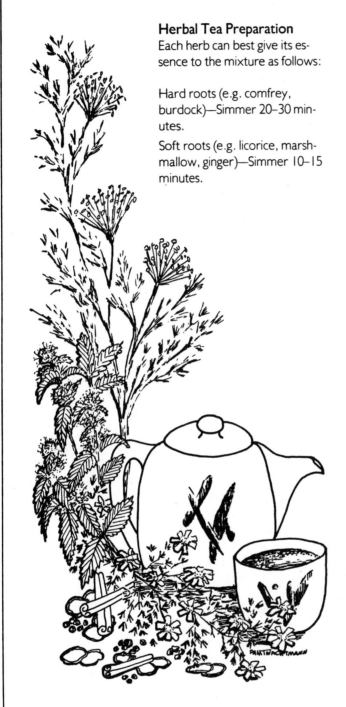

Summary

Winter is the coldest and darkest of seasons. It is the time when living creatures go within, while nature's crops are in storage. Nature and mankind are dominated by the *yin* principle. You must stay warm and it is important in winter especially to have a cozy spot to relax, sleep, and dream. Winter is the time of quiet preparation while awaiting the greening rebirth of spring with the rising winds, singing birds, and blooming flowers.

The winter season relates to the Water element and to the kidneys and bladder. These organs determine the water, mineral, and acid-base balances in the body by filtering the blood, making urine, and eliminating unneeded substances.

In the Chinese system, the kidneys control the life force energy; our vitality and longevity is said to be stored in the kidneys, visible externally by the sparkle or vibrancy of our eyes. Weak kidney energy may be experienced as lethargy or low energy and low vitality, while strong kidney energy may express the opposite, plus willpower and ambition, also ruled by the kidneys.

The *Nei Ching* says, "the kidneys are like the officials who do energetic work, and they excel in their ability and cleverness." This ability and cleverness may be strengthened by nourishing the receptive (*yin*) principle, of which the kidneys are part, through deep relaxation and reflection. From this process a blending of the inner with the outer can occur, which can give rise to knowledge, wisdom, and clear guidance.

The kidneys and Water element rule over the emotions. Both water and the emotions are unpredictable. When flowing, all is well; but when blocked or stagnant, great pressure can develop or disease can set in.

Kidneys, Water, and emotions are all ruled by the *yin* principle, the moon, the deep and dark. These aspects may stimulate fear from within, the emotion governed by the Water element, and fear or lack of faith may injure the kidneys or create an imbalance of Water in the body. With attunement to this "feminine" power, deep strength and wisdom develop. *Fear, ear,* and *hear* are all associated with the Water element; the ability to listen before acting is important to the well-being of this element.

The winter diet should be warming and substantial, with more whole grains, less fruit, lots of steamed or baked vegetables, and more dairy and flesh foods if these are in your diet. Soups are wonderful during the colder weather. Ocean foods like fresh fish and the seaweeds are especially good now. Soybeans, one of the complete vegetable proteins, is a good food with many uses, whether sprouted or cooked, as soy-milk and tofu; or fermented and aged to make miso.

Winter is a good time to do indoor exercises. Throughout the year, it is important to balance outward, energy-expanding activities like walking, jogging, tennis, and swimming, with quiet energy-accumulating, internally rejuvenating practices like yoga, tai chi, and breathing-relaxation. Keeping your spine and other joints flexible and mobile is important to how you feel. These practices can keep you young and vital.

Much of nature is hiding in her roots during winter, gathering the energy to be reborn in the spring. This gathering of energy is important to us as well, and we may facilitate it by brewing herbal roots and drinking lots of good tea. Ginseng root is a fine general tonic and rejuvenator, but burdock, comfrey, ginger, licorice, and sarsaparilla roots are also traditional energizers.

Vitally important to your health in winter, as in all seasons, is a balancing of the intake and output of your energy in the form of foods, feelings, and work. You need proper rest and sleep, relaxation and play, to balance the activity, stress, and work in your life. Creating and maintaining cleanliness within and without is also important to staying healthy.

The coming of each new season brings stress and change; illness can more easily overtake you then. But illness itself gives you the opportunity to re-evaluate your life. However, if you do this voluntarily and change with the new season you may prevent illness. Winter is an important time to feel what your inner changes are and weave them into your dance of existence.

冬

Winter

ELEMENT
DIRECTION
WATER
COLOR
NORTH
BLUE, BLACK
CLIMATE
COLD
QUALITY
STORAGE
EMOTION
FEAR
SENSE-ORGAN
EARS HEARING
SOUND
GROAN
FLUID
URINE
TASTE
SALTY
HAIR ON HEAD
INDICATOR
SMELL
PUTRID
BONES
TISSUE
KIDNEYS
BLADDER
YIN - ORGANS - YANG

in-balance	*imbalance*
keep warm	overactive
stay quiet	late nights and parties
sleep well	lack of rest and sleep
be at home	dissipation
look within	frustration
preserving—giving	hoarding

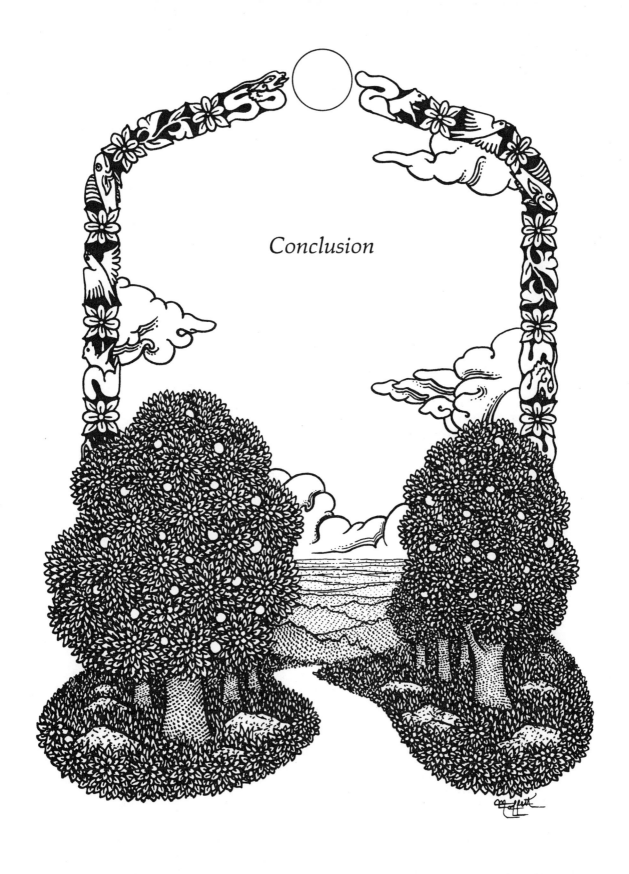

Conclusion

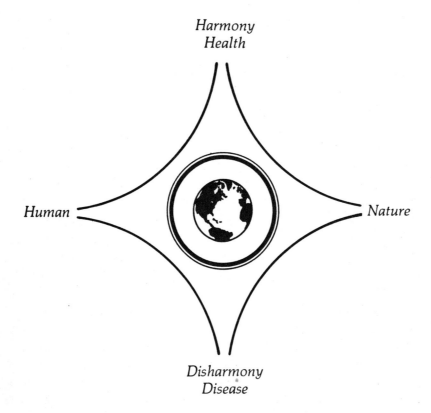

Harmony
Health

Human

Nature

Disharmony
Disease

Conclusion

Review

The main purpose of this book is to integrate several systems of medicine to create a whole approach to prevention and health care for you as an individual. Your well-being depends upon understanding and integrating your own cycles with those of nature. The ability to change and to adapt to each moment is what makes the human species a strong organism.

The "Basics" section sets forth the Chinese model of health and illness, in which the central idea is harmony between *yin* and *yang*, your inner and outer worlds. The traditional Chinese system is beautiful in its simplicity: by taking care to balance the *yin* and *yang* elements in your lives and adapting to the changing seasons, you can attain and maintain health.

The Chinese medical classic, the *Nei Ching*, tells us that long ago when people did not live by the laws of nature, they succumbed to illness and lived only half of their 100 years, rather like contemporary Western man. Western, or allopathic, medicine's role is to step in at this point with the heroics of saving and remedying those who have gone beyond their natural limits. Its diagnosis and treatment are defined in terms of the rational, linear aspects of existence, ignoring the roles of sensitive compassion and the intuitive understanding of the deeper mental, emotional, or lifestyle problems which go along with illness. The Oriental system, Tao (the way), which teaches right living and the Western system, which is concerned with very sick people, can work together. Both must be able to diagnose and treat conditions, understand human nature, and educate people in how to prevent illness. We must start supporting and nurturing each other more for staying well and less for getting sick. The compassion and special care that people receive when they become ill, and the release from having to go to school or to work can help support illness. Let us hope our culture will soon allot more money for education in self-care and for a deeper, more humanistic study of the habits and lifestyles which promote health. Workers might get health days from work and students play days from school, while insurance companies might pay for health checkups and preventive treatment like acupuncture and massage, and sponsor exercise and stress-reduction/relaxation classes. The whole system could work to keep people healthy. Many providers of health care know this and are shifting their focus to educate more patients to take responsibility for their own health.

The changes brought by each season correlate well with the Chinese Five Element theory. Each element is important for specific body organs, which in turn become especially vulnerable with each new season.

Season	Element	Organs
Spring	Wood	Liver, Gall Bladder
Summer	Fire	Heart, Circulation-Sex, Small Intestine, Three Heater
Late Summer	Earth	Spleen, Stomach
Autumn	Metal	Lungs, Large Intestine
Winter	Water	Kidneys, Bladder

Nutrition, exercise, and herbology help us adapt to the changing seasons and their different climates. In each section of the book one or more associated topics are discussed: cleansing diets and home-grown sprouts are important for a healthy spring; exercise and the heart for summer; good digestion, nutrition, and centering for late summer; easy elimination, cold prevention and the balance of meditation for autumn; and the receptive principle, reproductive processes, and warming nutrition for winter.

What is it that no one can live without, and that everyone wants more of? It is *energy*, both physical and mental. We spend time, dollars, and energy itself looking for it. Your life force ("chi" or "prana") depends on sunlight, clean air, pure water, good food, and sleep. The highest life force comes from unsullied nature, eating as close to the garden as possible while the sun, air, and water are still circulating in your food. Smaller quantities of good quality foods help you more than gorging on lower quality foods. Foods are fuels which heat the body, and balance your activity with the heat or coldness of each season. I do not feel the quality of animal foods is as good for you as the vegetable world's, but this choice is up to each individual's discretion and wisdom. Overeating or eating when upset affects your vital energy as much as eating poor foods. Eating light, wholesome foods prepared with love in a comfortable setting will nourish you completely.

Your life force needs to keep flowing through work, exercise, and clear emotional expression. Regular exercise is particularly important since many of us no longer live by physical labor. Each season has a form of exercise which is most appropriate for it, but all require moving the body toward its limits. Our personalities are expressed in the way we exercise, which in turn affects how we live. For example, a desire to express aggression, strength, and an ambition to win with the gratification of team play may lead you to choose an active, competitive sport like football, soccer, or hockey. Inner strength, independence, and stamina, are expressed through competitive sports like track and field, speed-skating, gymnastics, or skiing. Non-competition, relaxation, flexibility, and inner peace, emerge from the practice of yoga, tai chi, or ballet. A combined program is an important synthesis. Finding a balance of exercises to suit your needs and personality is as necessary as finding a good diet to meet your body's requirements.

Herbs can help you maintain your health as well as provide useful home remedies. Herbal effects are the basis for both traditional folk medicine and modern pharmaceutical formulas. But herbs in their natural form have fewer side effects when used correctly. Growing and gathering herbs, and making herbal teas, oils, salves, and other medicinals are activities that are becoming more and more popular. Growing your own herb garden depends on a clear understanding of both the plant's cycles and the changes each season brings to the earth. The *Nei Ching* states, "Planting and begetting are in accord

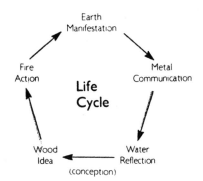

Earth
Manifestation

Fire
Action

**Life
Cycle**

Metal
Communication

Wood
Idea

Water
Reflection

(conception)

with the Spring, growing and cultivating are in accord with Summer; gathering in the harvest is in accord with Fall, and storing of the crop is in accord with Winter. If people habitually neglect to follow these rules, then the work of Heaven and Earth and the four seasons will be impeded."

Your own cycles of experience begin, grow, and mature and produce a harvest which is stored within, helping to give form to your next cycle in turn. Just as each season can be associated with a specific element, each element likewise relates to a certain life process.

The analogies are never-ending. Nothing is separate; everything is connected. Life is one continuous connection.

What is the Essence of Healing?

My own cycle over the last seven years has been centered around the question, "What s the essence of *healing?*" I feel much gratitude for the chance to develop a new understanding. My own growing and healing process is expressed throughout this book. I hope that you can use it in your own life, and that it may be helpful in your own learning and growth.

There are as many different healing systems as there are healing practitioners and cultures. What works for some doesn't work for others. And every culture has its own traditional and alternative approaches. Even techniques differ between practitioners; while one practitioner may have wonderful results with a specific system, another may not. Why is this? What causes healing to take place? There's no simple answer, yet I believe the *interchange of energy* between healer and healee is at the crux of the miracle of healing.

Healing has always been said to be an art, intrinsically intuitive. The healer must believe in what he or she is doing. Great practitioners have found equally remarkable results with Western medicine, herbalism, naturopathy, homeopathy, and acupuncture. The more open and ready the recipient is to be healed, the stronger tends to be the effect. A belief in the approach used and the ill person's trust in the healer are both critical. A deeper feeling for the physical, mental, emotional and especially the spiritual existence of the patient seems to make the successful healer rather than a simple equation of this treatment for that problem. If the healer can address the intrinsic healing power of the individual, improvement will be more likely to follow. The body must heal itself, even in the most technological modern medicine.

The continuum of illness and health is a manifestation of the continuum between confusion and clarity, and going from ill health to getting well involves growth and change. Often it is your pain or illness which guides you through the door of discovery and gets you in tune with your inner self. Becoming aware of past and current habits of carrying tension, and productive self-expression all seem to be essential in restoring your well-being.

The different systems of Western medicine, Chinese medicine, naturopathy, and homeopathy all bring light to bear on what it is that gives us health or illness, as well as the nature of the healing process.

Western medicine focuses primarily on the diagnosis and treatment of disease, but has become increasingly concerned with how lifestyle can cause illness. Physicians have been telling people for many years that if they stopped smoking, drank less alcohol, used less salt and sugar, lost weight, ate a moderate and balanced diet, exercised more, avoided extreme climates, and learned how to handle better the stress in their lives, they would be much healthier. If people as well as their physicians actually followed these and many other common sense rules, they could prevent much illness.

The Chinese tell us that there is an energy circulating through the body which should be kept flowing and in balance, in order to stay healthy. Illness arises when the flow of energy either stagnates or becomes excessively *yin* or *yang*, creating in turn an imbalance of the Five Elements. The causes of disease are described as the internal devils (emotions) and the external devils (climates). The Chinese describe also other internal causes of illness as stress, overeating, excess sexual activity, and overexertion, while external causes also include accidents, environmental pollutants, poisons, and microorganisms. Perverse climates and emotions will weaken us unless we protect ourselves. Each type of weather extreme affects specific organs, and may create immediate illness.

> *Wind can injure Liver (Wood)*
> *Heat can injure Heart (Fire)*
> *Humidity can injure Spleen (Earth)*
> *Dampness can injure Lungs (Metal)*
> *Coldness can injure Kidneys (Water)*

In the same manner, if emotions either get out of hand or are bottled up deep inside, they can create illness.

> *Anger can injure Liver*
> *Excessive joy or sadness can injure Heart*
> *Compulsion/Compassion can injure Spleen*
> *Worry/Grief can injure Lungs*
> *Fear can injure Kidneys*

The Chinese say that *yang* people tend to get *yang* diseases. These illnesses are hot, like fever, more superficial in the body, and active in that they are quick to change. They are often associated with pain or tension. Some examples of *yang* problems are inflammatory illnesses like skin boils, strep throat with fever, muscle pains, or diseases like hypertension. People who are too *yin* get *yin* diseases, commonly those of the deep organs or bones, whose weakened functions are harder to treat. They last longer and are accompanied by low energy. Examples are tuberculosis, hepatitis, and congestive heart failure. *Yang* diseases are more apt to surface during the *yang* seasons of spring and summer, while *yin* problems more often occur in the *yin* times of autumn and winter.

Traditional Chinese treatment corrects the energy imbalances through acupuncture and herbs. Acupuncture helps to restore the flow of energy by treating specific points. It strengthens and tones areas which are weak or deficient and drains or sedates areas or organs which are too strong or congested. Through the pulse reading of the twelve energy meridians at the radial (wrist) arteries (six positions, three superficial and three deep on each artery), the acupuncturist diagnoses the imbalance and checks the effectiveness of treatment. Herbs can similarly strengthen and relax certain organs and systems. Both acupuncture and herbs may take a while to work just as it has often taken months or years for the imbalance to manifest itself as disease.

The *Nei Ching* describes how health and longevity are affected by one's harmony with the *yin* (Earth), the *yang* (Heaven), and the seasons:

"Man draws life from Earth, but his fate depends upon Heaven. Heaven and Earth unite to bestow life-giving vigor as well as destiny upon man.
Man has the ability to conform to the four seasons. Heaven

and Earth act as his father and mother. He who is aware of the (needs) of all human beings is called the Son of Heaven.

For Heaven there exists Yin (the female element, darkness) and Yang (the male element, light); for man there are the twelve divisions of time (externally the twelve months and internally the twelve pairs of energy vessels). Heaven has cold and heat; man has (the abstract and the concrete,) the hollow and the solid.

One can take as invariable rule: Heaven and Earth; the changes between Yin and Yang; the infallibility of the four seasons; the knowledge of the methods of the twelve divisions of time. Not even imperial wisdom can take advantage of them or oppress them."

In *Rays of the Dawn*, by Thurman Fleet, the four naturopathic laws for harmony of the body, mind, and soul are set forth. First is the *law of nourishment*. He advocates combining mostly cleansing fruits and vegetables, along with a few building foods like grains, seeds, beans, nuts, dairy, and flesh, and a few lubricators (oils and butter), while avoiding congesting foods (all sweets and starches). The second is the *law of movement*. "Movement, or exercise is the only distributing agent of the body. Move every movable joint every day in every way that it will move until tiredness sets in. If pain develops in a joint, do not continue movement past that point, and it (the pain) will gradually subside." By moving to this point each day, soon the pain will disappear and the joints will become flexible and open. The third *law of recuperation* lists rest, recreation, and sleep as an important balance for activity. Fourth is the *law of sanitation*. "Cleanliness both inside and outside is indispensable in keeping the body healthy, wholesome, and beautiful, as well as the confines of the mind, soul, and spirit." Fleet refers to cleanliness in our diet, our environment, and proper bathing and elimination. If cleanliness is next to godliness, we may evolve to high planes of existence only in an environment and body that is clean and pure. These four laws suggest that the old-fashioned idea of balance and moderation in all things are keys for our well-being.

Homeopathy, a traditional system of medicine, was founded by Samuel Hahneman, M.D., and employs four important patterns of healing, known as Herring's "Law of Cure." As healing takes place in the mind/body, symptoms change in a given order: 1) they move from the center of the body toward the surface, 2) from the top of the body toward the bottom, 3) from more important organs to less important (for example from kidney to bladder to urethra), 4) symptoms reoccur or disappear in an order which is the reverse of their historical appearance.

These laws can be experienced as you watch your own healing. Take a deep belly breath and relax to see what is happening within you and to sense what you still need for your own treatment/healing. Breathing shallowly serves to insulate your mind from feelings or pain; just taking a few deep breaths allows frustrations, tensions, and emotions to surface and you feel better for it, more relaxed with clearer body and mind.

Everyday—breathe for life!

Being a health practitioner is not easy. Illness is often worrisome and frightening, and the physician/healer must bring comfort and emotional support to the patient. Diagnosis and treatment are not enough; there must be loving concern and education as well. But the responsibility is up to the patient to follow through the treatment and incorporate new understanding about prevention into daily life. Physicians often don't have the time to explain everything or provide the needed reassurance and comfort, and patients often don't want to know too much, or more importantly, do not want to take an active role in becoming healthy. Your happiness and health do not come from someone outside you; you are your own best doctor. Illness often means a turning point in your life and growth which is usually positive. After you get over the anxiety about being sick, you may find new insights into yourself and your life.

Edward Bach, M.B., B.S., D.P.H., English healing practitioner and creator of the Bach Flower remedies, believes that illness is a spirit-body disharmony. Illness offers a chance to grow, according to *Heal Thyself:*

"Let it be briefly stated that disease, though apparently so cruel, is in itself beneficial and for our good and if rightly interpreted, it will guide us to our essential faults. If properly treated it will be the cause of the removal of those faults and leave us better and greater than before. Suffering is a corrective to point out a lesson which by other means we have failed to grasp, and never can it be eradicated until that lesson is learnt. Let it also be known that in those who understand and are able to read the significance of premonitory symptoms

A doctor's role is as a servant to people's needs, growth, and knowledge; but he or she cannot be a slave to people's unwillingness to improve themselves.

disease may be prevented before its onset or aborted in its earlier stages if the proper corrective spiritual and mental efforts be undertaken. Nor need any case despair, however severe, for the fact that the individual is still granted physical life indicates that the Soul who rules is not without hope."

Harmony of spirit and matter is essential to bringing about a healing process affecting ourselves, our families and eventually the whole earth. Our era, our lives, our planet, all certainly need a cleansing and refinement as well as a new balance of earth and spirit. As individuals, we can help bring about this cleansing by reducing our own intake of chemicals and other toxins; of synthesized foods; and of diets heavy in flesh, eggs and milk products; and by replacing these with a lighter, more natural diet of cleansing fruits and vegetables, whole grains, nuts, beans, seeds, and sprouts; and by drinking uncontaminated spring water. And being out in nature whenever possible replenishes our spirits as well.

A continuous process of cleansing, building, and creativity will bring us clarity and strength, so that we can clear out all that is in the way of our becoming self-realized, aware of our true selves. This means becoming conscious of *who we are, what we are doing here,* and *doing it*—there is nothing else, nowhere else—only *here and now.*

So then, *What is the essence of healing?*

Truth
  Faith
    Communication
      Understanding
      Love
          are all important!

Change is the essence of healing.

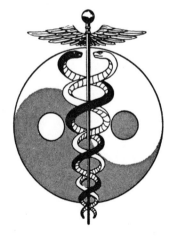

Health Report Card

Go through each item on the report card and grade yourself. Basically, the grade will be your feeling of satisfaction or unhappiness with your situation about the particular item.

A sample grading scale might be:

BIG SMILE, TEETH SHOWING (1)   REALLY HAPPY WITH YOURSELF

NICE SMILE (2)   SATISFIED

JUST LIPS (3)   OKAY; NOT GOOD, NOT BAD

FROWN (4)   DISSATISFIED; COULD REALLY IMPROVE

GRAVE STATE (5)   IT'S KILLING ME

You may wish to use your own grading scale such as 1 to 5. Check the Key after the report card for explanations concerning each item you are grading Have fun!

Subject	Grade	Subject	Grade
General Diet	_____	*General Cleanliness*	_____
Diet Awareness	_____	Appearance	_____
Eating Mood	_____	Skin, Hair, Nails	_____
Eating Habits	_____	Teeth	_____
Willpower	_____	Intestines	_____
Natural Foods	_____		
Animal Foods	_____	*Cycles*	_____
Processed Foods	_____	Physical	_____
Chemicals in Diet	_____	Mental	_____
		Emotional	_____
General Activity	_____	Menstrual	_____
General Energy Level	_____		
Balance with Intake	_____	*General Health*	☐
Daily Exercise	_____	*Attitude*	☐
Exercise Discipline	_____	*Health Improvement*	☐
Breathing	_____	*Desire for Health*	☐
		Improvement	
Rest	_____	*Health Knowledge*	☐
Relaxation Ability	_____		
Quality of Sleep	_____		
Dreams	_____		

Report Card Key

General Diet	How do you feel about your overall diet and eating habits?
Diet Awareness	What do you put into your body? Do you care? Do you get the best foods you can? Without chemicals and additives? Do you take the time to prepare food and to eat, or is it something you do passing through?
Eating Mood	Do you eat in a pleasant setting? Do you relax before eating? Do you eat when emotionally upset?

Eating Habits	Do you chew your food well? Do you breathe well while eating? Do you overeat or eat before bed?
Willpower	Are you in control of your eating or is food in control of you?
Natural Foods	Do you feel you eat enough fresh foods in your diet, i.e., fruits, vegetables? Do these and other foods that come to you as nature grows them, i.e., nuts, beans, seeds and whole grains, comprise the major part of your diet?
Animal Foods	Do you eat many animal products? Does this feel good to you?
Processed Foods	Do you eat packaged, quick snack foods?
Chemicals	Do you eat foods preserved with substances that are not naturally found in nature or the body?
General Activity	Does it seem appropriate to you?
General Energy Level	Are you happy with the amount you have through the day?
Balance with Intake	Do you put out as much as the fuel you take in? How is your efficiency?
Daily Exercise	Yes? No? Does it feel good to you?
Exercise Discipline	Can you keep up an exercise program?
Breathing	Do you breathe deeply?
Rest	Do you get enough rest to keep yourself well and functioning optimally?
Relaxation Ability	Are you capable of relaxing yourself? Is it hard to clear away daily stresses?
Quality of Sleep	Do you sleep well? Do you fall asleep easily? Are you well rested upon arising?
Dreams	Are you often aware that you have dreamed? Do you try to remember and write your dreams down? Do you learn from them?
General Cleanliness	Do you keep your environment and your body clean? Could you do better?
Appearance	Are you happy with how you present yourself?
Skin, Hair, Nails	Do you brush or clean them regularly?
Teeth	Do you brush and floss after eating? Daily? Rarely?
Intestines	Do your bowels move well and regularly? Do you often feel congested or get constipated?
Cycles	Are you aware of cycles that you have? Are you in touch with being on and off sometimes when engaged in certain activities? Do you have accidents?

Physical	Are you aware of a physical energy cycle? Does your energy vary over a day, a month, a year? Are you able to go inward and rest when needed, or are you more likely to resist and become ill?
Mental	Are you aware of changes in alertness and your thinking abilities? Do you use this awareness advantageously?
Emotional	Are you aware of mood changes, ups and downs? Do you have periods of crankiness or other emotions surfacing? If needed, can you become more or less sociable at your will? Do you get lonely?
Menstrual	Women, are your periods regular and comfortable? Men, are you aware of your cycles, especially cleansing times?
General Health	How do you rate your overall health?
Attitude	Are you happy about your health? About yourself, your life? Do you spend time alone? Do you get bored easily?
Health Improvement	Has your health improved in the last year?
Desire for Health	Are you willing to work at improving it?
Health Knowledge	Do you have sufficient knowledge to live and grow in your environment, i.e., to improve you health?

If you used the point system of grading, the following scale will be of interest to you:

Total score	*Status*
35–55	Remarkable health habits
55–80	Good care; you should stay healthy
80–110	Average; step it up
110–135	Poor habits; could really improve
135–	Terrible—how do you feel?

Personal Health History

date_____

I. *General Information*

Name_____phone (   )_____

Address (mailing) _____birthdate_____

City, State, Zip _____birthplace_____

Work/occupation _____

Breast or bottle fed (circle)   home or hospital birth (circle)

Approximate date of last medical exam _____

Are you presently under a doctor's care?_____ Who? _____

for what? _____

Do you currently take any medications? What? _____

Rx _____

Non Rx_____

Are there any other healers, helpers, or therapies with which you are involved?

Who and/or what? _____

_____How long?_____

II *Focus*

What is your chief concern?_____

_____

What are your goals for your health/life? _____

_____

List any other current symptoms or problems _____

_____

_____

What are three factors in your life that seem most important to your daily health? _____

_____

_____

III. *Review of Systems/Symptoms*

Mark a check (✓) by problem if you have, or have had it occasionally in recent years. Mark two checks (✓ ✓) if problem occurs often; and three checks (✓ ✓ ✓) if it is a regular difficulty.

_____weight loss or gain

_____fatigue

_____confusion

_____nervousness

_____muscle tension

_____muscle cramps

_____cold hands and/ or feet

_____itching

_____skin rashes

_____skin boils

_____headaches

_____fevers

_____nightmares

_____dizziness

_____blackouts

_____ringing in ears

_____earaches

_____double or blurry vision

_____eyestrain

_____nasal congestion

_____sinus pressure

_____nosebleeds

_____mucous problems

_____sores in mouth

_____tongue problems

_____coated tongue

_____bad breath

_____sore throats

_____teeth or gum problems

_____neck pains

_____cough

_____difficulty breathing

_____shortness of breath

_____coughing blood

_____heart palpitations

_____chest pains

_____breast lumps or pains

_____poor endurance

_____gas

_____abdominal pains

_____difficult digestion

_____constipation

_____diarrhea

_____hemorrhoids

_____urinary problems

_____burning on urination

_____bladder or kidney infection

_____bedwetting

_____blood in urine

_____back pains

_____leg swelling

_____bone or joint pains

_____arm, shoulder, or leg problems

_____joint swellings

_____bruise easily

_____irregular bowel movements

_____bloody or black stools

_____number BMs daily

_____increased sexual desire

_____decreased sexual desire

_____birth control

_____aging rapidly

IV. *Women*

date of last menstrual period _____

are your periods regular?_____frequency? _____

how many days is your flow? _____

painful or symptomatic periods? _____

when was your last pap test? _____

number of pregnancies_____deliveries _____

    abortions_____miscarriage_____other _____

do you practice birth control? _____

    what form? _____

check forms you have practiced and write years practiced:

BC pills _____ rhythm _____

IUD _____ mucous method _____

diaphragm_____ astrological_____

chemical spermicides _____ condoms _____

_____ abstinence _____

List your children:

Name	Sex	Birthdate
_____	_____	_____
_____	_____	_____
_____	_____	_____

V. *Past Medical History*

Do you have allergies? _____

If so, to which medicines? _____

to which foods? _____

or to what in the environment? _____

_____

Do you take any regular medications, either prescribed or over-the-counter?
What and how often? _____ _____

_____

_____

Do you take any regular vitamin, mineral, or herbal supplements? Please list _____

_____

_____

Have you had any operations? What and when (year)? _____

_____

_____

Any major injuries/accidents? What? _____

_____

Any major illnesses or hospitalizations? What and when? _____

_____

_____

Check any of these you have incurred. Write approximate year.

____pneumonia	____high blood pressure	____kidney infection
____tuberculosis	____low blood pressure	____parasites
____hepatitis	____heart disease	____rheumatic fever
____asthma	____heart attack	____measles, german
____diabetes	____cancer	____measles, regular
____hypoglycemia	____blood transfusion	____mumps
____epilepsy	____migraine headache	____chicken pox
____eczema	____ulcer	____polio
____skin boils	____anemia	____whooping cough
____kidney stone	____arthritis	____diptheria
____drug reaction	____obesity	____colitis
____psoriasis	____mental breakdown	____syphilis
____hives	____jaundice	____gonorrhea

VI. *Family History*

List birthdates and health status of immediate family. Write A/W if they are alive and well. Write in any chronic illness(es) they have, or if deceased, mark D and write the cause.

relationship	*birthdate*	*health*
mother	_____	_____
father	_____	_____
sister(s)	_____	_____
	_____	_____
brother(s)	_____	_____
	_____	_____

Do any of these illnesses run in the family? Who?

____diabetes	____cancer
____high blood pressure	____epilepsy
____heart disease	____mental illness
____tuberculosis	____thyroid problems
____asthma	____obesity
____gout	____twins (not illness)

VII. *Diet and Exercise*

Do you have a good appetite? _____

good eating habits? _____

How do you feel about the foods you eat? _____

_____

_____

Do you floss your teeth/mouth regularly? _____

Write the percentages in your diet of these food categories. Total 100

fruits_____   grains_____   dairy_____

vegetables_____   nuts, beans, seeds_____   meats_____

What percent of your diet is raw_____cooked_____? Total 100

What percent of your dairy foods is raw_____pasteurized_____? Total 100

List the percents of these meat categories. Total 100

beef_____   chicken_____   fish_____   Other_____

Do you use foods made with chemical additives or preservatives? _____

What? _____

What percent of your food is from restaurants? _____

What percent of your food do you prepare yourself? _____

For the next categories, write the average number of times in a week these items are consumed in your diet.

(e.g. 0 = never, 2/w = twice weekly, 3/d = three times daily)

fried foods _____	alcohol _____
white or brown sugar_____	beer _____wine _____
food additives (chemicals) _____	liquor_____
_____	drugs _____
coffee_____	what?_____
nicotine _____	freq? _____

Is there one or more particular food flavors that you crave? (circle) sweet, salty, spicy, bitter, sour, other?

Do you have a garden? _____vegetable_____flower_____

Do you enjoy exercise? _____mild?_____strenuous?_____

How often do you exercise weekly? _____

Do you sweat easily? _____ How often? _____

List exercise and frequency.

_____   _____

_____   _____

_____   _____

Do you have any pets? What? _____

VIII. *General Questions*

Are you able to express your emotions/feelings? _____

_____

Is there any you feel predominantly? _____

anger_____ sadness_____ fear_____ sympathy/worry _____

excessive joy_____ depression_____ other _____

Are you too emotional or too unemotional? _____

What makes you nervous? _____

_____

Is there much stress in your life? _____

If so, what does it surround? i.e. family, work, finances, relationships, etc. _____

_____

Do you sleep well? _____ How many hours/night? _____

Do you dream? _____ How often? _____

Do you remember any?_____ Are they helpful?_____

Are you happy with your general energy level? _____

Is there a low point in your day?_____ When? _____

Do you have a favorite time of the day? _____

Do you have a favorite climate/weather? What? _____

Are there climates you especially don't like? What and why? _____

_____

What is your favorite color(s)?_____

What is your favorite season? _____

What level did you complete in school? _____

Any other organized life/trade training? _____

What, if any, was your military service? _____

With whom do you live? _____

    relationships? _____

What is your work? _____

What are your hobbies/pleasures? _____

_____

_____

What are your indulgences? How often? _____

_____

_____

Have you ever abstained from or "quit" anything? _____

What and why? _____

For how long? _____

Do you ever crave that which you have curbed? _____

When? _____

How do you feel about yourself? _____

_____

About your life? _____

_____

Appendix: Health and Astrology

I HAVE FOUND ASTROLOGY USEFUL both in my everyday life and in my medical work with others, particularly as it relates to character and personality types, human psychology, and interpersonal relationships. The study of astrology stimulates one's intuitive sense. In our observation of the cycles of nature, we observe and sense our own cycles. A study of these cycles may help us to learn more about ourselves and create greater harmony in our lives.

Astrology has existed for so long and is still actively shared in our society via newspapers, books, and radio and TV that we can consider it to have some validity. But neither the newspaper predictions nor the scientific viewpoint of astrology as a Dark Age superstition give a true understanding of its value.

Astrology is a dualistic science. One side deals objectively with astronomical data, that is, the regular, timed movement of the planets through space. The Earth's spin creates our days; its path around the Sun creates our seasons and years. The Moon's relationship to the Earth creates our months. Time—in the linear, rational sense—is thus based on this aspect of astrology.

The other side of astrology is conceived more subjectively and intuitively from the effect that these cycles of solar, lunar, and planetary movement have upon nature, animal, and human life. Just as the basic concepts of traditional Chinese medicine connect Heaven and Earth with humans and nature, astrological philosophy joins the daily earthly life with the universal activities. We are all contained in this "greater whole," and we may experience peace when we incorporate this greater realm within our humble selves. If nature is affected by these planetary cycles, and we are influenced by nature, then we must be connected to the astrological patterns.

Astrology and medicine were once unified. Hippocrates, the father of modern medicine, wrote that he used them together. Knowledge of astrology was needed to make accurate diagnoses and he even claimed that a physician was a fool if he did not use astrology. Illnesses were seen as disharmony between the physical body and extraterrestrial influences, based on the natural laws of the universe.

Galen, likewise, applied astrology to medicine, and in *De Metodo Medicine* he said, "the state of the sky, the season of the year and region or country should be considered in diagnosing and treating human ills." Carl G. Jung studied, used, and wrote of astrology in relation to psychology and understanding the human organism. He called astrology scientific intuition, "whose postulates were based on centuries of experience, recorded in the collective unconscious." In *Psychology and Alchemy*, Dr. Jung wrote, "Science began with the stars, and mankind discovered in them the dominants of the unconscious, the 'gods' as well as the curious psychological qualities of the zodiac; a complete projected theory of human character."

Astrology and Chinese Medicine

There are many correlations between astrology and Chinese medicine. The Sun and Moon are the dominant influences upon the Earth and they represent the male-active and female-receptive principles respectively, the conscious and unconscious, day's light and night's darkness, or the *yang* (Sun) and *yin* (Moon) principles. The movement of the Earth around the Sun creates the light and dark cycle of the seasons. (Summer—most *yang*, Winter—most *yin*).

The number twelve is a key, representing totalities. The twelve months make one year. The twelve signs of the zodiac create a complete cycle of experience. The Chinese lunar years number 12; thus 12 years, each represented by a certain animal—such as rooster, tiger, pig—describes a full cycle.

Both the Chinese year and the zodiacal year start with the birth of spring, the time of beginnings in nature. Aries, March 21–April 19, has been considered the first sign of the zodiac.

The four elements of astrology are Fire, Earth, Air and Water. A correlation between these elements and the Chinese Five Elements is easily seen.

The twelve signs of the zodiac from Aries to Pisces go consecutively Fire, Earth, Air, and Water so that each element describes three astrological signs. One is termed cardinal (initiating), another fixed (maintaining), and the last mutable (adapting).

The Chinese System states that Fire creates Earth which creates Metal (Air) which creates Water, and Water creates Wood or helps plants to grow. The meanings of these elements are similar in both systems.

The Chinese Fire element relates to activity, warmth, and maturation as it is the most *yang* element and rules the hot summertime and the organs of heart and small intestine. The astrological Fire signs are all considered active, masculine or *yang*, and hot and passionate types. Aries combines mental and physical activity as it rules the head, brain, and nervous system; Leo rules the heart, spine, motor nerves and is concerned with circulation of blood, with electricity, and with movement; and Sagittarius, another warm and social, active positive *yang* sign rules the hips.

The Chinese Earth element governs the late summer and transition times and the stomach, spleen and digestive processes in the body. It relates to material, stability, and the ability to focus and to manifest. The Earth signs of the zodiac are considered receptive or *yin*, concerned with form and feeling (sensing). The astrological Earth element also gives practicality, stability, and concern for earthly matters. Taurus, the first Earth sign, rules the neck, and is geared toward material and possessions, permanency, and security. Virgo seeks more mental stability, analyzing and focusing on the world of the mind. Virgo rules the intestines and digestion and assimilation. Capricorn rules the knees and bones, the stable and supporting body structures. Capricorn relates to business and to hard work, especially using Earth materials like wood, stone, and soil—as in building and gardening.

The Air element corresponds to the mind—ideas, knowledge, and communication—and relates to the Chinese Metal element which has similar attributes—mind, thinking, and communication. The Metal element is dominant in autumn, the time of school, work, and new ideas; it rules the lungs and large intestine in the body. Proper breathing and elimination of wastes is important to clear thinking. The three Air signs of ideas, travel, and communication are Gemini, Libra, and Aquarius. Gemini likewise rules the lungs, and all forms of communication and education like writing, music, and art. Libra seeks mental balance and communication between people as in partnerships, contracts, and all relationships. Libra rules the kidneys, an organ of elimination of waters, and body chemistry balance. Aquarius, full of ideas and knowledge, both day-to-day and universal, rules the ankles and carries the water (the essence) of life.

The Chinese Water element—the element that is the most *yin*—is dominant in winter and corresponds to feelings, nurturing, and reflection, the process between communication and creation. The Water element rules the kidneys and bladder, which oversee and balance the body's water. The three Water signs are considered receptive or *yin,* and are guided by their feelings and senses. Cancer is a nurturing sign relating to the home, motherhood, and expression of feelings. It rules the breasts and womb, both important to child rearing. Scorpio is known as a more intense sign of deep feelings and desires and rules the genitals and sexuality. Pisces, a water sign, governing the feet, is sensitive, both bodily and spiritually. The Water element of both systems and the Water signs are concerned with the subconscious mind and the dream world.

The Wood element, the additional one of the Chinese Five elements comes between the Water and Fire elements. It corresponds to the life forms, the plants and the human body which needs the four other elements to exist: Fire, the Sun to give light, warmth and growth; Earth, soil for support and to provide nourishment; Air for the breath of life; and Water for circulation of its needs. As the Chinese describe the Wood element, it has equal aspects of each of the other four elements. It relates the organizing, planning, and overseeing functions in one's body and in one's life, and thus it includes the reflection or the "taking a look at" aspect of the Water element, the projected action on ideas and incorporation of intuition of the Fire element, the Earth element's ability to focus and organize, and, of course, the thinking and communication gifts of the Metal or Air element.

Above all, these elements and their interrelationships create and allow change and growth. All cycles, including the seasons, the Chinese Five Elements, the astrology, and your body's, may help enhance your health and vitality when you learn to know and use them.

Birth Charts

When we are born, the planets are in a specific configuration. The position of each planet within the zodiac has a certain set of characteristics, influences, or possibilities. What is manifested is a specific map, a guideline to personality, goals, and potentials.

The astrology that is available to most of us, as in the daily forecasts in newspapers or monthly predictions found in some magazines, is based on our birthday, our Sun sign only. Sun sign astrology is useful but limited because we are many things and represent all parts of the zodiac. We are ever changing through the year and throughout our lives, the change dependent upon the influences which dominate and on where we focus our energies. The Moon has a strong effect, especially on women, as do the rising sign (the sign that is on the horizon at the time of birth) and the position of the other planets. The Moon rules over the subconscious and our emotional world, the rising sign signifies our personality or how we appear to other people. Each planet has certain characteristics and influences.

The birth chart is divided into twelve parts, called the *houses.* Each is 30° of the 360° zodiac circle and two hours of a 24-hour day. Each house represents a certain sign, specific aspects of one's life, a feeling, and certain parts of the body. For example, the first house relates to Aries, the head and awareness of the self, the "I am" sense. The sixth house of Virgo corresponds to service and health, the intestines and the function of assimilation.

The movements of the celestial bodies, their progressions, and their connection with our birth charts are called the *transits.* The angles between the planets in our birth chart or that occur during transits are called *aspects* and can create potential for harmony or conflict. These angles such as 0° (conjunction), 60° (trine), 90° (square), or 180° (opposite) can cause attraction or repulsion, and thus compatibility or incompatibility. In reading someone's astrological birth chart, one must take into consideration the whole while looking at the sum of its parts.

The Astrology Cycle

The twelve signs of the zodiac act essentially as the totality of all possible experiences in the universe. No one sign is "better" than another, they are all needed to make the whole. People with strong accentuations to certain signs will show certain characteristics, attitudes, or even body types. The Sun, for example, represents our basic purpose and potential. A brief overview of the Sun signs will show their interconnections within the complete cycle.

Aries is the first sign, signifying the pure spirit (energy) entering the body, creating the force of springtime, like a plant arising from the Earth. Taurus is pure substance, receiving the energy of Aries. As builders working with the materials of the Earth, Taurus brings stability and permanency. Gemini balances the force with the object, creating motion; and it relates to the mind and intellect, travel and communication. Cancer is the personalizing sign adding emotions to the mental world of Gemini. Sensitive Cancer, the universal womb, allows the birth of the Individual Man (Leo) from its waters of life linking the four primitive signs (Aries–Cancer) to the four individual ones (Leo–Scorpio).

Leo is the spirit of creation made manifest, solar fire to matter. Proud Leo, aware of the self, predominantly seeks to express creative abilities. Virgo, the Individual Woman, is the medium for creative self-expression. Virgo is organized and discriminatory and takes care of details. Libra is the balance between Ideal Man and Woman joining in the ideal relationship, the marriage of spirit and matter. Libra seeks harmony through cooperation and compromise. Scorpio, the second water sign, one of emotional power, prepares for a new manifestation. As it deals with death and rebirth, it is the transition from the individual signs to the universal ones (Sagittarius–Pisces).

Aspiring toward illumination, Sagittarius, the first of the signs focusing on universal values, seeks the meaning of life through active experience and the higher philosophies. Able and organized, Capricorn is a creative Earth sign dealing with the practical use of materials toward the spiritual upliftment of humankind. Friendly Aquarius is the fixed Air sign of ideas, knowledge, and friends, and attempts to bridge the relationship between the self and the universe. Pisces is the dissolution, the separation of boundaries and limits, the blending of all forms. The last Water sign is the link between the end of one cycle and the beginning of another.

Biorhythms

The cycles that exist in our solar system are the keys to understanding and using astrology in our lives. These cycles are regular and consistent and reveal, when we become aware of them, the patterns that exist on the Earth and within each of us. Our regular body cycles are termed *biorhythms*.

The organs, especially the hormone glands, have specific cycles, regular patterns of hormone production and release. For example, the adrenal gland, which releases metabolic hormones as well as adrenalin, gives us our active energy. It is most active in the early morning about 8 A.M. but takes a low ebb about 4 P.M., a time often associated with sluggishness and irritability.

The scientific concept of biorhythms claims that we each have certain regular cycles for our physical, mental, and emotional states, as well as more subtle cycles such as self-awareness, appreciation of beauty, and the sense of spirituality. The physical cycle is 23 days, emotional is 28 days (lunar), and the mental one is 33 days. These start in waves going from outward states (being active, mentally clear and emotionally expressive) to the more internal awareness (being less physically active, less sharp in the mind, and emotionally withdrawn), then more outward again.

These cycles do not necessarily all occur together, but have a constant interplay. The times when each shifts from outward to inward, or from inward to outward are considered stress or crucial days and are times to be more careful. These days have been shown to correlate more commonly with accidents and illnesses.

The lunar cycle is important, particularly to women as it influences their hormonal and menstrual cycle. This 28-day rhythm also influences men, especially night energy, dreams, and their emotional nature. The Moon cycle is crucial to the process of fertility and creativity. As the Moon is our nightly reflector of sunlight, it is our monthly *yin-yang* cycle. Being aware of the lunar stages and their effect on us is also important to staying healthy.

Each planet has a complete cycle which is its time to revolve around the Sun. Saturn, for example, changes signs each 2 1/2 years and its full cycle is 29 years. Thus, the important "Saturn return," a time often filled with learning, allows us the time to take a deep look at our lives, reevaluate, and go forward. It occurs at ages 29, 58, and 87. Uranus, the planet of revolution and changing beliefs changes signs every seven years and completes its full cycle every 84 years.

Other planets have their effects as well: Mercury rules over our mental world; Venus over our romantic, artistic side; and Mars stimulates our physical energy and adventure in the world. Saturn has an important influence on our growth and learning the universal laws, while Jupiter is the benevolent father of the zodiac giving and supporting our spiritual nature. The outer planets, Uranus, Neptune, and Pluto may well have a lesser action on our everyday lives, though a stronger one on the universal level and on our more subtle energies. And who knows? Many feel there is one more planet yet to be discovered in our solar system.

Astro-Biochemistry

There is a system called *astro-biochemistry*, which combines both astrology, the study of celestial influences upon people, and biochemistry, "the chemistry of life." It has been in use about 80 years since George Washington Carey, a noted biochemist of the early 1900s, allocated the body's twelve basic mineral salts to the twelve signs of the zodiac. These inorganic mineral salts, also called tissue or cell salts, were isolated and produced by Dr. William Scheussler, whose name is still associated with many homeopathic medicines, most importantly these twelve common tissue salts. When Dr. Carey organized these with the zodiac, it gave another dimension to their use.

These salts, such as sodium chloride, calcium phosphate, and potassium sulfate, are the inorganic constituents of foods which help to form blood and body tissues and nourish the cells. They are called cell or tissue salts as they are cell and tissue builders. The organic parts of foods are substances with a carbon element base such as albumen, oils, fibrin, etc., and are digested in the stomach and intestines to be used by the body as fuel and heat, and in such functions as breathing, circulation, and digestion.

The inorganic mineral salts, prepared homeopathically as small white tablets on a milk sugar base, can be taken as supplements to the diet, and are in the same form as those found in foods, and thus, readily absorbed and used. The 6X potency is most commonly recommended.

These tissue salts can be used individually for nourishment and for balancing the body on a cellular level to create greater harmony. With a clean, relaxed, and well-working system, we can extract from foods all that our body needs for daily use. However, if we become deficient via excessive activities or stress, or poor digestion and assimilation, we may need supplementation.

Astro-biochemistry's role is to make use of these mineral salts to balance the body and prevent illness depending on one's astrological makeup and current planetary influences. Some examples of salts a person might need include one's Sun sign salt, the sign opposite the Sun sign which may be weak, the Moon or rising sign's salt, or the salt of a sign in which there is an affliction (adverse angles).

The importance of mineral salt balance is pointed out by Dr. Charles W. Littlefield, an analytical chemist in the following quote from *The Zodiac and the Salts of Salvation:*

The twelve mineral salts are, in a very special sense, the material basis of the organs and tissues of the body and are absolutely essential to their integrity of structural and functional activity. Experiments prove that various tissue cells will rapidly disintegrate in the absence of the proper proportion of these salts in the circulatory fluid. Whereas the maintenance of this proportion insures healthy growth and perpetual renewal.

These mineral salts are, therefore, the physical basis of all healing. Regardless of the school employed, if these are absent from the blood and tissues, no permanent cure is possible.

Sign	Symbol		Character	Conscious Aim
Aries	♈	Ram	Independent Active	Leadership
Taurus	♉	Bull	Productive Determined	Security
Gemini	♊	Twins	Experiential Artistic	Establishment of relationships
Cancer	♋	Crab	Sensitive Imagination	Emotional enfoldment
Leo	♌	Lion	Playful Magnetic	Creative self-expression
Virgo	♍	Virgin	Mental Discriminating	Perfection
Libra	♎	Scales	Creative Musical	Harmony
Scorpio	♏	Scorpion	Secretive Intense	Power
Sagittarius	♐	Centaur	Optimistic Friendly	Wisdom
Capricorn	♑	Goat	Practical Ambitious	Integrity
Aquarius	♒	Water-Bearer	Universal Intellectual	Truth
Pisces	♓	Fish	Dreamer Compassionate	Understanding

Motto	Ruling Planet	House/Associations	Capacity For
I am	Mars	1st-Self-awareness Early environment	Self-assertiveness
I have	Venus	2nd-Possessions Money, Values	Determination
I think	Mercury	3rd-Communication Short travel	Versatility
I need	Moon	4th-Home Old age	Home life
I will	Sun	5th-Children Self	Affection
I analyze	Mercury	6th-Service Health	Discrimination
I balance	Venus	7th-Marriage Arts	Partnership
I desire	Pluto	8th-Birth and death Occultism	Secret forces of nature
I see	Jupiter	9th-Philosophy Long travel	Aspiration
I use	Saturn	10th-Careers Honors	Business
I know	Uranus	11th-Friends, Social Life Hopes & wishes	Altruism
I believe	Neptune	12th-Institutions Destiny (Karma)	Super-physical

Planet	Symbol	Cycle**	Character	Body Associations
Sun*	☉	—	Male, light, warmth, purpose, will, conscious, creative, growth, activity	Energy, heart, spine
Moon	☽	29 days***	Female, receptive, fertile, cycles, emotion, instinct, imagination, subconscious	Womb, stomach, breasts
Mercury	☿	88 days	Mind, communication, travel, thought, child	Brain, nervous system
Venus	♀	225 days	Romance, arts, beauty, social elements, family	Veins, venous system
Earth	⊕	365 days	Stability, productive, realism, form	Whole body
Mars	♂	687 days	Action, initiating, aggression, war, courage, passion, adventure, sex	Solar plexus, muscular system, sexual organs
Jupiter	♃	12 years	Higher mind, philosophy, law, good fortune, expansion, hope	Liver, gallbladder, pancreas
Saturn	♄	29 years	Teacher, cosmic law, karma, time, limitation, lessons	Bones, teeth, ligaments
Uranus	♅	84 years	Beliefs, revolution, enlightenment, inventions, electronics, ESP	Pituitary, spinal fluid, aura
Neptune	♆	165 years	Subconscious, oceans, dreams, drugs, ideals	Pineal, arterial blood
Pluto	♇	248 years	Underworld, death, dark, cold, rebirth, transformation	Pineal, adrenals, kidneys

*Not a planet   **One revolution around the Sun   ***Around the earth

Cell Salts Allocated to the Signs of the Zodiac

Aries	Kali Phosphoricum (Potassium Phosphate)	K_2HPO_4
Taurus	Natrum Sulphuricum (Sodium Sulphate)	NA_2SO_4
Gemini	Kali Muriaticum (Potassium Chloride)	KCl
Cancer	Calcarea Fluoricum (Calcium Fluoride)	CaF_2
Leo	Magnesia Phosphorica (Magnesium Phosphate)	$Mg_3(PO_4)_2$
Virgo	Kali Sulphuricum (Potassium Sulphate)	K_2SO_4
Libra	Natrum Phosphoricum (Sodium Phosphate)	NA_2HPO_4
Scorpio	Calcarea Sulphurica (Calcium Sulphate)	$Ca_3(SO_4)_2$
Sagittarius	Silicea (Silica Oxide)	SiO_2
Capricorn	Calcarea Phosphorica (Calcium Phosphate)	$CA_3(PO_4)_2$
Aquarius	Natrium Muriaticum (Sodium Chloride)	$NACl$
Pisces	Ferrum Phosphoricum (Iron Phosphate)	$FePO_4$

Herb Glossary

Alterative—a general term referring to a substance which can alter or change a bodily condition by restoring normal bodily functions, e.g., goldenseal root, burdock root, sarsaparilla root, sassafras bark, yarrow, red clover flowers.

Annual—a plant whose whole cycle from seed to death occurs within one year, e.g., garlic, pennyroyal, sunflower.

Anodyne—a substance which relieves pain, e.g., coca leaf, hops, opium, mullein flower.

Anthelmintic—a substance which expels or kills intestinal worms, e.g., wormwood herb, pumpkin seed, white oak bark.

Antiemetic—a substance that relieves nausea and vomiting, e.g., clove, opium, peppermint, warm water, lavender.

Antipyretic—a substance which reduces or prevents fever, also called febrifuge and refrigerants, e.g., aspirin, alcohol sponging, birch bark, cold bath, dandelion, feverfew, wintergreen, yarrow, chamomile, sage.

Antiseptic—a substance that inhibits the growth of microorganisms in living tissue, e.g., hydrogen peroxide, myrrh, witch hazel herb.

Antispasmodic—a substance which reduces or prevents muscular spasms or cramps, e.g., lobelia herb, chamomile, marijuana, valerian root, cramp bark, skullcap, mullein leaf.

Aperient—a gentle laxative agent, e.g., licorice root, coffee bean.

Aromatic—an herb with a spicy, pungent taste yet pleasant and fragrant smell, e.g., lavender, rose, chamomile.

Astringent—a substance which causes the contraction of tissues helping to check the discharge of oils, mucus, and fluids, e.g., lemon, alum root, wild sage leaves, oak barks, pomegranate, cranesbill root.

Bark—the outer covering of stalk, tree, or root.

Biennial—a plant which takes two seasons (two years) for its complete cycle, e.g., parsley, fennel, mullein.

Bitter(tonics)—a substance with an astrigent, acrid or disagreeable taste which stimulates flow of saliva and gastric juices, the digestive process, and the appetite, e.g., mugwort, wormwood, chamomile, dandelion root, goldenseal root, hops flowers, blackberry leaf.

Carminative—a substance which helps to reduce and eliminate gas from the stomach and intestines, e.g., fennel seed, anise seed, chamomile, cinnamon, cayenne, peppermint, catnip, ginger root, cardamom, caraway, coriander and cumin seeds.

Catarrh—an inflammation of any mucous membrane, most often the respiratory tract, causing congestion and secretion of mucus. Agents helpful are salt water, borage, goldenseal, red sage, vitamin C.

Cathartic—a substance causing the evacuation of the bowels, also laxative or purgative, e.g., aloe, castor oil, cascara sagrada, buckthorn bark, senna leaves, rhubarb root, figs, prunes, psyllium seed.

Decoction—a preparation made by simmering an herb or part of an herb in water for a period of 30 minutes or more. Usually the harder parts of plants like the root, bark or seed are used in an approximate proportion of one ounce per pint of water.

Demulcent—a substance which, when taken internally, will soothe inflamed mucous membranes or prevent them from irritation, e.g., comfrey root, slippery elm bark, fenugreek seed, plantain leaf, mullein leaf, flaxseed, egg white, honey, licorice root, marshmallow root, olive oil, oatmeal, coltsfoot leaf.

Diaphoretic—a substance which induces sweating when taken internally, e.g., bonset herb, yarrow herb, elder flowers, chamomile, pennyroyal, ginger root, hyssop leaf.

Disinfectant—a substance which cleans an area of debris and lowers the number of microorganisms, e.g., air, fire, bleach, sun, myrrh.

Diuretic—a substance which increases the flow of urine, e.g., uva ursi, parsley, cornsilk, leeks, juniper berries, cleavers herb, dandelion, water, horsetail grass, cubeb berries.

Emetic—a substance which induces vomiting, e.g., lobelia herb, ipecacuanha root (ipecac), mustard seed, foxglove.

Emmenagogue—a substance which promotes menstrual flow, e.g., pennyroyal herb, tansy herb, rue herb, blue cohosh root, wormwood.

Emollient—a substance which when used externally on the skin or on mucous membranes acts to soften or protect, e.g., slippery elm bark, oils, cocoa butter, comfrey root, glycerin, marshmallow leaf/root, flaxseed meal, oatmeal.

Expectorant—a substance which helps to loosen and expel mucus from the respiratory tract, e.g. hyssop herb, garlic, yerba santa leaf, wild cherry bark, comfrey root, elecampane root, mullein leaf, licorice root, wild sage leaf, coltsfoot leaf, slippery elm bark.

Extract—a solution which contains the essence from the plant, usually in a greater strength. Decoctions, infusions and tinctures are examples.

Flower—the part of a plant containing the reproductive organs which are often surrounded with brightly colored petals.

Fruit—any plant products, usually edible and containing the seed(s), pulp, or pit. As in fruits, vegetables, grains.

Hemostatic—a substance that slows or stops bleeding, e.g., comfrey root, alum root, goldenseal root, lemon juice, capsicum.

Hepatic—a substance which affects the liver, e.g., dandelion root, wild yam root, barberry root.

Herbology—the study of plants, trees, shrubs or their parts used in medicine.

Infusion—the extraction of the properties of a substance by soaking (steeping) it in water. The most common method of preparation for herbs is as a tea (infusion).

Laxative—a substance which produces a gentle action upon the bowels, e.g., cascara sagrada, dandelion, coffee, Oregon grape root.

Medicinal—any substance used to treat disease.

Mucilaginous—mucus-like, referring to a substance which swells and forms a slimy mass in water, used to soothe inflamed areas, e.g., slippery elm bark.

Nervine—a substance which calms and/or strengthens the nerves, e.g., valerian root, catnip, chamomile, hops, linden flower, skullcap, rosemary, celery, passion flower, nerveroot.

Nephritic—a substance useful for the kidneys, e.g., uva ursi leaf, buchu leaf, juniper berry, nettle, oatstraw.

Pectoral—a substance used to treat problems of the chest and lungs, e.g., mallows, mullein, elecampane, comfrey, garlic.

Perennial—a plant which continues its cycle of growth for more than two years, e.g., peppermint, comfrey, ginseng, rosemary, trees and shrubs.

Poultice—a substance heated and applied to an irritated or wounded area or the skin for comfort or remedy, e.g., comfrey leaf or root, flaxseed, slippery elm bark.

Purgative—a strong acting laxative/cathartic, used to relieve constipation by stimulating bowel activity, e.g., senna leaf, buckthorn bark, aloe, rhubarb root.

Restorative—a substance which increases a person's vitality or vigor, e.g., foti tieng, ginseng root, gotu kola, sarsaparilla root.

Root—the part of a plant usually below ground that holds it in place, draws water and nourishment from the soil, and stores food.

Sedative—a substance which calms the nerves, relieves excitement and nervousness, e.g., valerian root, chamomile, peach leaf, skullcap, catnip.

Seed—the part of a plant which will grow, containing the embryo and the capacity to develop into new plant if sown.

Sialogogue—a substance which increases the flow of saliva, e.g., capsicum, ginger root, cubeb berries, jaborandi leaf, mustard.

Specific—a substance which has a certain effect in a particular disease.

Steep—allowing substances to infuse into water, most commonly after water has been boiled and poured over them, to extract their essence.

Stimulant—a substance which quickens and enhances the functional activity of the body, e.g., dandelion root, coffee, guarana, kola nuts, black teas, ginseng root, rosemary leaf, nutmeg, damiana leaf, fennel seed, caraway seed, capsicum (cayenne).

Stomachic—a substance which gives strength or tone to the stomach or stimulates the appetite by promoting digestive secretions, e.g., ginger, cardamom, chamomile, cumin, lavender, lemon, thyme, sage, yarrow.

Styptic—an agent which helps to stop bleeding.

Tea—an infusion made by pouring boiling water over a substance(s) and letting it steep in a covered container.

Tincture—an alcoholic solution of a medicinal substance.

Tonic—a substance that improves body tone, invigorates, restores and strengthens the total body or specific systems, e.g., ginger root, golden seal root, raspberry leaf, skullcap, valerian root, vervain, comfrey, elecampane, capsicum, kelp, ginseng root.

Vermifuge—a substance that destroys or expels intestinal worms, also anthelmintic, e.g., wormwood, white oak bark, bitter root, vervain.

Vulnerary—a substance helpful in healing wounds, e.g., plantain leaf, speedwell, burdock, self-heal, comfrey, chlorophyll.

Bibliography

Ardell, Donald B., *High Level Wellness: An Alternative to Doctors, Drugs, and Disease.* Emmaus, Pennsylvania: Rodale Press, 1972.

ArgIsle, Bethany S., *That Healing Feeling.* Fairfax, California: KeyWhole Publishing, 1981.

Bach, Edward, *Heal Thyself: An Explanation of the Real Cause and Cure of Disease.* London: C.W. Daniel Company, 1976.

Burroughs, Stanley, *The Master Cleanser.* Kailua, Hawaii: Burroughs, 1976.

———, *Healing for the Age of Enlightenment.* Kailua, Hawaii: Burroughs, 1976.

Carey, George Washington, and Inez Eudora Perry, *The Zodiac and the Salts of Salvation.* New York: Samuel Weiser, Inc., 1977.

Chaffee, Ellen E., and Esther M. Greisheimer, *Basic Physiology and Anatomy.* Philadelphia: Lippincott Company, 1969.

Christopher, John R., *Dr. Christopher's Three Day Cleansing Program and Mucusless Diet.* Provo, Utah: Christopher, 1978.

Connelly, Dianne M., *Traditional Acupuncture: The Law of the Five Elements.* Columbia, Maryland: Center for Traditional Acupuncture Inc., 1979.

Cooper, Kenneth H., M.D., M.P.H., *The New Aerobics.* New York: Bantam Books, 1978.

Davison, Ronald, C., *Astrology.* New York: Arc Books, 1970.

Denniston, Denise, and Peter McWilliams, *The TM Book: How to Enjoy the Rest of Your Life.* New York: Warner Books, 1975.

Dinger, J. E., *Leaves of Gold.* Williamsport, Pennsylvania: Coslett Publishing.

Dufty, William, *Sugar Blues.* New York: Warner Books, 1976.

Feng, Gia-Fu, and Jane English, *Lao Tsu: Tao Teaching.* New York: Vintage Books, 1972.

Feng, Gia-Fu, and Jerome Kirk, *Tai Chi—A Way of Centering and I Ching.* New York: Collier Books, 1976.

Fleet, Thurman, *Rays of the Dawn.* San Antonio, Texas: Concept Therapy Institute, 1950.

Ganong, William F., *Review of Medical Physiology*. Los Altos, California: Lange Medical Publications, 1969.

Garrison, Omar V., *Medical Astrology*. New York: University Books, 1977.

Goodman, Louis S., and Alfred Gilman, *The Pharmacological Basis of Therapeutics*. New York: Macmillan Company, 1967.

Hittleman, Richard, *Richard Hittleman's Yoga: 28-Day Exercise Plan*. New York: Bantam, 1978.

Hsu, Lee, trans., *Basic Acupuncture Techniques*. San Francisco: Basic Medicine Books, 1973.

Hylton, William, ed., *Rodale Herb Book*. Emmaus, Pennsylvania: Rodale Press, 1974.

Iyengar, D.K.S., *Light on Yoga*. New York: Schocken Books, 1976.

Joy, Brugh, M.D., *Joy's Way: A Map for the Transformational Journey*. Los Angeles: J.P. Tarcher, 1979.

Kloss, Jethro, *Back to Eden*. New York: Beneficial Books, 1972.

Kulvinskas, Viktoras, *Sprout for the Love of Every Body*. Wethersfield, Connecticut: Omango Press, 1978.

Lane, Alice, *Guide to Cell Salts and Astro-Biochemistry*. New York: Zebra Books, 1975.

Leonard, Jon N., J. L. Hofer, and N. Pritikin, *Live Longer Now*. New York: Grosset and Dunlap, 1974.

Mann, Felix, *Acupuncture: The Ancient Chinese Art of Healing*. New York: Vintage Books, 1972.

Menzies, Rob, *The Herbal Dinner*. Millbrae, California: Celestial Arts, 1977.

Muhr, Elaine, *Herbs*. Eugene, Oregon: Muhr, 1974.

Muir, Ada, *The Healing Herbs of the Zodiac*. St. Paul, Minnesota: Llewellyn Publications, 1974.

Muramoto, Naboru, *Healing Ourselves*. New York: Swan House, 1973.

Nutrition Research, Inc., *Nutrition Almanac*. New York: McGraw-Hill Book Co., 1979.

Ornstein, Robert E., *The Nature of Human Consciousness: A Book of Readings*. New York: Viking Press, 1973.

Price, Weston, *Nutrition and Physical Degeneration: A Comparison of Primitive Diets and Their Effect*. La Mesa, California: Price-Pottenger Nutrition Foundation, 1948.

Roberts, Toni M., Kathleen McIntosh Tinker, and Donald W. Kemper, *Health-Wise Handbook*. Garden City, New York: Doubleday, 1979.

Rose, Jeanne, *Herbs and Things*. New York: Grosset and Dunlap, 1979.

Rosenblum, Arthur, *The Natural Birth Control Book*. Philadelphia: Aquarian Research Foundation, 1977.

Sakurazawa, Nyoti, *You Are All Sanpaku* (English version by William Dufty). New York: Award Books, 1969.

Shelton, Herbert M., *Food Combining Made Easy*. San Antonio, Texas: Dr. Shelton's Health School, 1976.

Shook, Dr. Edward E., *Elementary Treatise in Herbology*. Lakemont, Georgia: CSA Press, 1974.

Stone, Dr. Randolph, *Health Building: The Conscious Art of Living Well*. Ambolu, India: The Tribune, 1962.

Szekely, Edmond Bordeaux, *The Ecological Health Garden*. Costa Rica: International Biogenic Society, 1978.

Timms, Moira, and Zachariah Zar, *Natural Sources: B-17 and Laetrile*. Millbrae, California: Celestial Arts, 1978.

Veith, Ilza, *Nei Ching: The Yellow Emperor's Classic of Internal Medicine.* Berkeley, California: University of California, 1972.

Wallnofer, Heinrich and Anna von Rottauscher, *Chinese Folk Medicine and Acupuncture* (translated by Marion Palmedo). New York: Crown Publishing, 1965.

Whittlesay, Marietta, *Killer Salt.* New York: Avon Books, 1977.

Wigmore, Ann, *Naturama: Living Textbook.* Boston: Hippocrates Health Institute.

Index

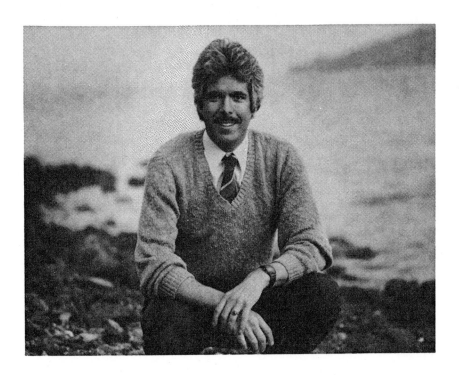

Dr. Elson M. Haas is an innovative and active practitioner in the fields of nutritional and preventive medicine. He directs an "integrated" general practice at the Marin Clinic of Preventive Medicine and Health Education in San Rafael, California. Dr. Haas also practices in San Jose. His personal interests are in the areas of environmental and planetary healing and educating children. He is also the author of the *Seasonal Food Guide* and the new *Staying Healthy with Nutrition*.

Dr. Elson Haas is a partner with Bethany Argisle in Health Harvest Unlimited, Inc. a corporation that creates and distributes health educational products such as Sole-Sox™ (Reflexology socks), the Acupuncture T-shirt, the Chakra T-shirt, and other anatomy clothing. Write for a free catalogue:

Health Harvest Unltd., Inc.
P.O. Box 427
Fairfax, CA 94978

he doesn't draw you in, include you,
validate + encourage you. He piles
on shoulds + ↑ guilt about not doing
the right things. Too intellectual
yet not intellectually satisfying.
Lots of info - no Truth.
Doesn't ring true.

✓⚡✗

1   Intro to body + energy sys
    How it works
        SPLT vs KID
        ching vs sang

2+ Elements

later→ Emotions   being out of control
       6 Evils   really describing them

ACTION

<u>ACTION</u> CT to Earth

Tx for respons. for Earth

learned
passivity where are you drawn
go to your "power places"
to recharge + tune in to
the Earth + your part
in life on this planet.

_____

Write from inside out

How it feels inside

Not how it looks.

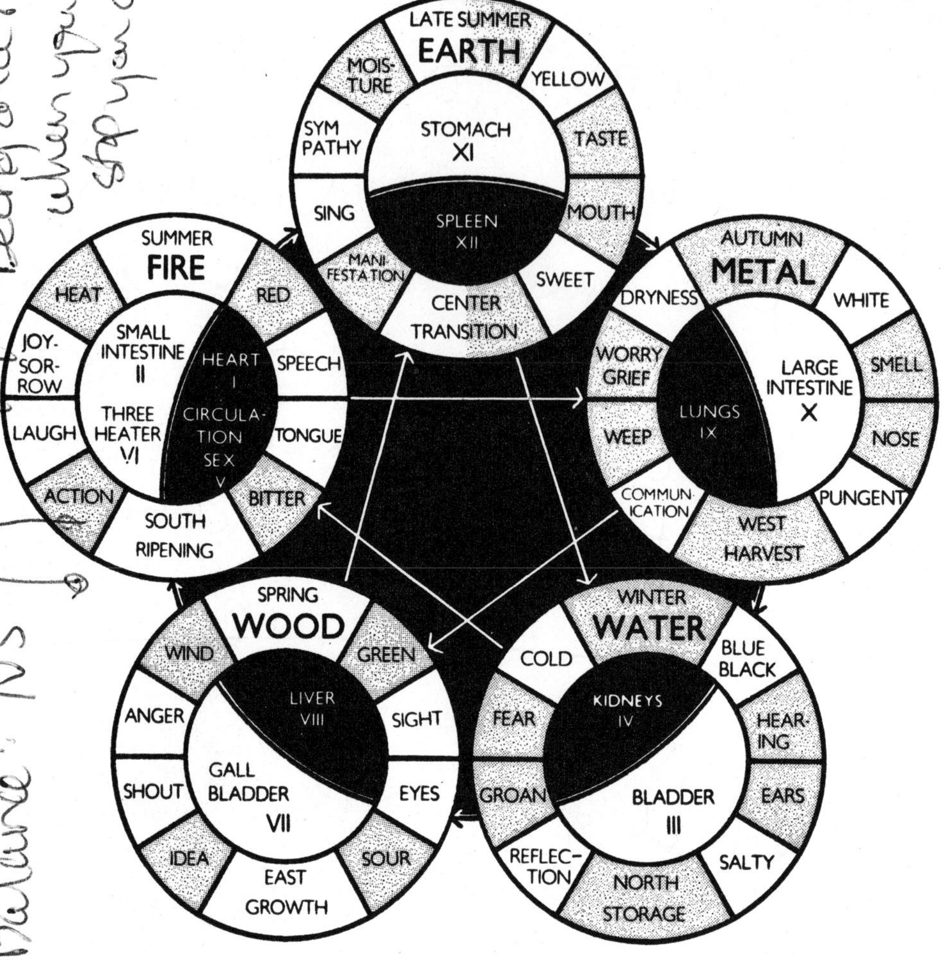

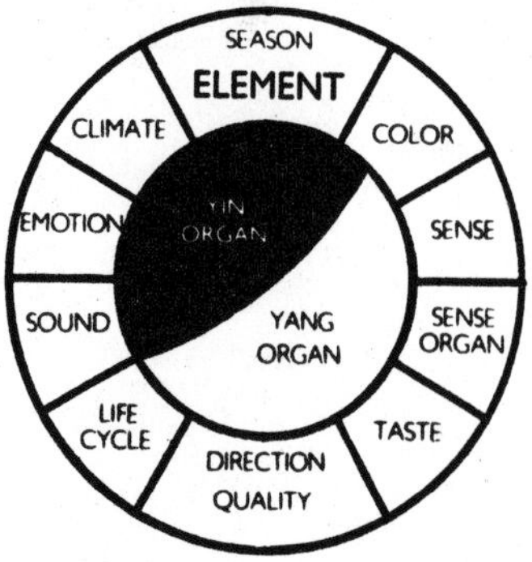

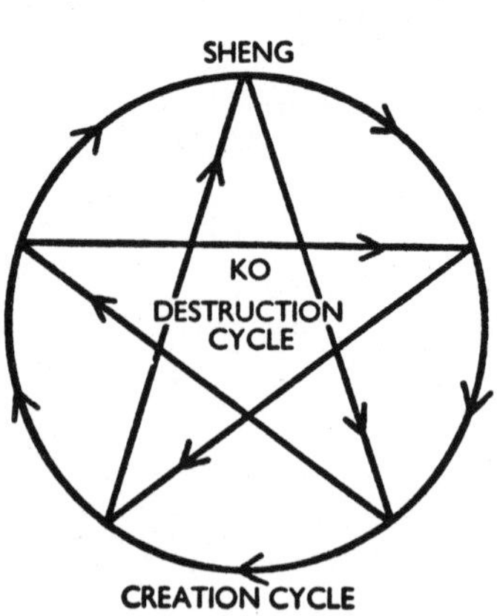

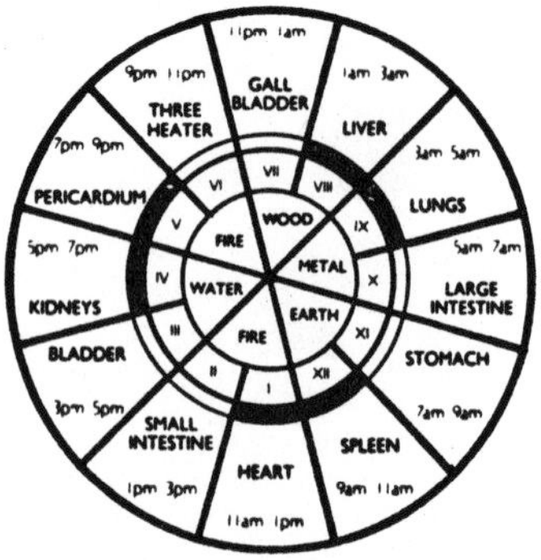

Better paper, larger cleaner type. Proper sentences structure. Grammar. Clear, concise, no B.S. Less words more info.

— Balance: NS — pulley sys. Being on a roll, when you finally stop you crash.